Barbara Sanches

Evaluation of the phagocytosis of CAE virus-infected macrophages

Barbara Sanches

Evaluation of the phagocytosis of CAE virus-infected macrophages

Against Corynebacterium pseudotuberculosis

ScienciaScripts

Imprint

Cover image: www.ingimage.com

This book is a translation from the original published under ISBN 978-3-330-99746-2.

Publisher:
Sciencia Scripts
is a trademark of
Dodo Books Indian Ocean Ltd. and OmniScriptum S.R.L publishing group

120 High Road, East Finchley, London, N2 9ED, United Kingdom
Str. Armeneasca 28/1, office 1, Chisinau MD-2012, Republic of Moldova, Europe
Managing Directors: Ieva Konstantinova, Victoria Ursu
info@omniscriptum.com

Printed at: see last page
ISBN: 978-620-8-62147-6

SUMMARY

CHAPTER 1

INTRODUCTION

The art of animal husbandry dates back to the Ancient Ages, around 7,000 years BC. In the Palaeolithic period (up to 26,000 years BC), primitive, nomadic man observed that the seeds that fell to the ground multiplied in a few months, making it unnecessary to go in search of food; instead, man began to set up small settlements, initiating rudimentary agriculture. In the Neolithic period (26,000 to 5,000 years BC), man began to improve agriculture with the use of ploughs and began domesticating animals, with the return, in addition to meat, being the supply of milk.

The goat, Capra hircus, was one of the first animals to be domesticated by man, around 7,000 years before Christ, having as ancestors the wild goat, Capra aegragus or Benzoar goat from eastern Asia and found to this day in the Mediterranean and Middle East, mainly on the island of Crete; the Capra falconiere from the Himalayas, and the Capra prisca from the Mediterranean basin. The domestication of the goat is such an ancient process and so fundamental to human life and history that it is mentioned in various literary sources, including the Bible.

As it is a docile animal and highly adaptable to different climatic and soil conditions, its breeding has spread to various regions of the world, making its products a source of food for many peoples, such as the Egyptians who used its milk to make dairy products, and the Mesopotamians, Hebrews and Palestinians who fed on the meat and milk of these animals.

Regional diversities were responsible for the emergence of goat breeds, which were improved over time, and in the modern era the appearance of small groups of animals is the result of man's selection of these animals.

Currently, goat farming is of great importance in the world's livestock industry and forms part of the livestock economy, being very widespread, especially in developing countries. According to FAO data (2005), the world population of goats and sheep is 1,886,980,000 head; Brazil ranks 16th among the world's goat and sheep herds. The top countries are China, with a herd of 183,207,008 head, India with a herd of 120,000,000 head and Pakistan with a herd of 54,700,000 head.

The preliminary results of the agricultural census carried out by the Brazilian Institute of Geography and Statistics (IBGE) in 2006 indicate a goat population of around 11,460,735 head, with the Northeast region accounting for 10.632,816 (92.78%) head, the South 260,441 (2.27%) head, the Southeast 272,238 (2.38%) head, the North 167,791 (1.46%) head and the Centre-West 127,449 (1.11%) head (ANUALPEC, 2006). Also, according to the IBGE agricultural census, in 1975 the goat population was around 6,709,428 head, in 1985 this population rose to 8,207,942 head and in 1995 it fell to 6,590,646 head, and today this figure exceeds 10 million head. These figures show that the activity has fluctuated over the last 25 years and that in the last ten years the herd has increased considerably.

Of the products that come from goat farming, milk, meat and skin deserve special mention, but the former is still the most widespread product, and the third most consumed milk in the world. However, according to the FAO, Brazil contributes 1.08 per cent of world production. This can be explained by the lack of proper management and health of the herd, the lack of knowledge about the physiology of reproduction and the nutritional requirements of these animals, and some diseases that lead to a drop in production and the discarding of animals from the herd, thus causing great economic damage directly to the producer and indirectly to the country's economy.

Two infectious diseases responsible for economic losses deserve to be highlighted: caprine encephalitis virus arthritis (CAV) and caseous lymphadenitis.

The first is caused by a virus from the Retroviridae family, genus Lentivirus, present in the majority of Brazilian herds, and is an enzootic disease that causes arthritis and leukoencephalomyelitis, and less frequently causes respiratory and mammary gland alterations (QUINN et al., 2005; AL-QUDAH et al., 2006).

The second is caused by the Gram-positive bacterium Corynebacterium pseudotuberculosis, a mesophilic bacillus that produces an exotoxin capable of hydrolysing lysophosphatidylcholine and sphingomyelin, resulting in the formation of abscesses in superficial or deep lymph nodes; it is considered a zoonosis (COSTA, 2002; DERCKSEN et al., 2000). Infection in humans is considered to be occasional and occupational in goat and sheep farmers, as well as in professionals linked to the breeding of these species, and can come from direct contact with purulent material from abscesses; ingesting raw milk is an important form of contagion for both humans and animals (RADOSTITIS et al., 1994; ÇETINKAYA et al., 2002).

Both diseases have a worldwide occurrence and their pathogenesis has not been fully elucidated, making it difficult to achieve successful eradication and control programmes. In addition, both the bacterium and the virus have a tropism for host macrophages, corroborating the hypothesis that the two diseases interfere with the host's innate response mechanisms, perhaps if they are associated.

CHAPTER 2

LITERATURE REVIEW

2.1 CAPRINE ENCEPHALITIS VIRUS ARTHRITIS

Caprine encephalitis virus arthritis (CEVA) is an infectious, multisystemic disease, insidious and chronic in nature, caused by a virus from the Retroviridae family, Orthoretrovirinae subfamily, Lentivirus genus (QUINN et al., 2005), which has a tropism for cells of the host's monocyte/macrophage lineage and affects goats of all ages, sexes and breeds (LEITE et al., 2004; LARA et al., 2005).

Among the viruses of this genus, we can mention human immunodeficiency virus (HIV), feline immunodeficiency virus (FIV), equine infectious anaemia virus (EIAV) and Maedi Visna virus (MVV), which are responsible for causing immunodeficiency-associated infections that develop slowly over months or years (QUINN et al., 2005; RAVAZZOLO et al., 2006).

Present in herds all over the world, epidemiological studies of the disease have been carried out in various countries. Thus, Al-Qudah et al. (2006) investigated the epidemiology of VAEC infection in Jordanian goats over a period of one year and concluded that 23.2 per cent of the herds studied were seroreagent, a higher figure when compared to the Turkish herd which reported 1.9 per cent of infected herds. In Central Mexico, the prevalence of VAEC was 28.6 per cent (TORRES-ACOSTA et al., 2003), in Australia 82 per cent (GREWAL et al., 1986), in Italy 38 per cent (GUFLER et al., 2007), in Quebec, Canada, 82.5 per cent (BELANGER; LEBOEUF, 1993) and in the United States 73 per cent (CUTLIP et al., 1992).

In Brazil, the AEC virus is widespread in the goat population and prevalence data differ according to the regions studied. In Rio de Janeiro, Cortez-Moreira et al. (2005) found that 14.1% of the samples analysed were reactive to agar gel immunodiffusion (AGID) and enzyme-linked immunosorbent assay (ELISA). In Ceará, in a study of 130 farms located in 30 municipalities, the prevalence of VAEC infection was 1% when studied as a whole, not differing between breeds and aptitudes, but the prevalence was higher when only dairy herds were analysed (4.6%), while in Pernambuco the prevalence was 17.6% (PINHEIRO et al., 2001) and in the state of São Paulo it was 29.8% (FERNANDES, 1997).

The AEC virus (VAEC) causes leukoencephalomyelitis, mainly observed in young animals, and persistent arthritis, chronic interstitial pneumonia, endurative interstitial mastitis and progressive weight loss in adult animals (BANKS et al., 1983; NARAYAN et al., 1985; LARA et al., 2005; AL-QUDAH et al., 2006). As a result, a drop in milk and meat production, and the death or discarding of seropositive animals from the herd are identified as the main factors in the damage caused by this disease (SILVA et al., 2001; LARA et al., 2005; LILENBAUM et al., 2007).

Transmission occurs horizontally, after ingesting milk or colostrum from goats infected with the virus (CRAWFORD; ADAMS, 1981; ADAMS et al., 1983; EAST et al., 1987), since the virus can be found in milk secretions as free particles or inside somatic milk cells (SMITH; SHERMAN, 1994). In a 2003 study on experimental infection with VAEC, Lara et al. investigated the forms of transmission and observed that all the animals tattooed with equipment contaminated with the virus showed persistent seroconversion, thus concluding that the indiscriminate and serial use of contaminated syringes, needles and tattooists are important sources of contamination and transmission of the virus.

Although there have been no reports of the disease in humans, Tesoro-Cruz et al. (2003) found antibodies against VAEC in children who had contact with goats or their products (milk, cheese, etc.), but did not find these same antibodies in children who had no contact with this animal species.

The diagnosis of AEC is based on the detection of serum antibodies to the AEC virus, with ELISA and IDGA being the most commonly used tests (LARA et al., 2003; CORTEZ-MOREIRA et al., 2005; ANDRÉS et al., 2005; BRINKHOF; VAN MAANEN, 2007). Other alternative and more sophisticated techniques such as Western blot and polymerase chain reaction (PCR) have not been widely accepted to date due to the complexity of the method and the difficulty in standardisation (KNOWLES JR et al., 1994; CORTEZ-MOREIRA et al., 2005; QUINN et al., 2005; BRINKHOF; VAN MAANEN, 2007).

Despite intensive studies, there is still no treatment for AEC and many animals remain asymptomatic, acting as reservoirs for the virus. Therefore, the disease must be controlled through segregation programmes. There is no effective vaccine (QUINN et al., 2005).

The exact pathogenesis of AEC has not been fully elucidated. The persistence of the virus in various organs and/or tissues despite an intense immune response is characteristic of lentiviruses (FLURI et al., 2006; RAVAZZOLO et al., 2006). This similarity between VAEC and HIV was reported by Zink et al. (1990) who described that both lentiviruses persist indefinitely and replicate productively in macrophages, causing encephalomyelitis, pneumonia and lymphadenopathy. This is due to a large number of viral transcripts in these tissues, suggesting an association between viral gene expression and the development of organ dysfunction.

VAEC and MVV, unlike other lentiviruses that infect lymphocytes, have a tropism for cells of the monocyte/macrophage lineage and dendritic cells (GENDELMAN et al., 1986; ZINK et al., 1990; QUINN et al., 2005; FLURI et al., 2006; RAVAZZOLO et al., 2006). However, immunological studies have shown that sheep infected with MVV in the terminal stages of the disease show an inversion of the proportions of CD4 T lymphocytes /$CD8^{++}$ in the peripheral blood and joints. Thus, it is possible that VAEC-infected goats may have impaired T helper lymphocyte function, similar to acquired immunodeficiency syndrome (AIDS) in humans (ZINK et al., 1990). Thus, animals with arthritis, when compared to asymptomatic animals, have a high viral load and high antibody titres (RAVAZZOLO et al., 2006) and a probable impaired proliferative activity of T helper cells. This is due to the fact that the production of cytokines is reduced or their production profile is altered as a result of the altered response of T helper cells, which play an indispensable role in setting up a solid immune response of cytotoxic T cells and memory B cells, thus impairing both the cellular response and the humoral response against the virus (FLURI et al., 2006).

Ravazzolo et al. (2006), in a study measuring viral load, distribution of the virus in the body, histopathological lesions and cytokine expression, observed that the expression of gamma-interferon (IFN-γ) varied independently of viral load in animals infected with VAEC. The role of IFN-γ in the immune response against VAEC remains to be fully elucidated. Somehow in various viral models this cytokine has an antiviral function stimulating both the innate immune response and the adaptive response; on the other hand, IFN-γ can activate viral transcription by binding to IFN-γ responsive elements present along the repetitive terminal chain of the VAEC genome. It is also well known that IFN-γ mediates viral activation in latently infected cells which can subsequently lead to the recognition and elimination of these cells by the immune system (LECHNER et al., 1997).

Interleukin (IL) 6 is highly expressed in AEC and has been shown to co-stimulate T lymphocytes and act as a factor in the differentiation of B cells (LECHNER et al., 1997).

IL-12 was also observed to be slightly elevated, perhaps due to an inadequate macrophage response. In T-cell stimulation, an increase in IL-4 suggests that it is antigen-specific, with no correlation with viral load (RAVAZZOLO et al., 2006).

Studies of VAEC replication in macrophages, in vitro, have shown that the expression of the viral genome is dependent on the state of maturation of the cells, i.e. the deoxyribonucleic acid (DNA) of the virus in monocytes is not transcribed until the cells become macrophages, and restricted viral replication is a mechanism that allows the virus to go undetected by the cells of the immune system for long periods (ZINK et al., 1990).

Lechner et al. (1997) reported that the change from predominantly Th1 to Th2 immune response could be related to the severity of arthritis. However, the expression of cytokines present in the study suggested that the definition of the immune response may be more complex. Because the synovial membrane and lymph node drainage contained cells expressing IFN-γ (a typical Th1 immune response cytokine) during acute infection (day 12) and in goats with severe clinical arthritis, they demonstrated that goats with clinical arthritis did not exhibit a deficiency in IFN-γ expression in response to VAEC. The expression of local IFN-γ mRNA depended more on viral transcription than on the stage of arthritis. However, preliminary studies indicated an increase in IL-10 expression (supporting the Th2 immune response) in the lymph nodes of goats with chronic arthritis. No IL-4 transcript was detected in the synovial fluid or lymph nodes of VAEC-infected animals. Therefore, considering the histological in situ hybridisation results obtained from the synovial membrane, it was difficult to classify goat arthritis as a Th1 or Th2 disease.

Wilkerson et al. (1995) reported that the alternative pathway of antigen presentation by macrophages and dendritic cells predominates over the classical pathway in perpetuating the production of memory antibodies, especially in a medium enriched with antibodies and low levels of antigens.

The role of cells of the monocyte-macrophage lineage in the context of this disease is important, as it is a cell related to innate immunity and also the target cell of the virus. Thus, Werling et al. (1993) observed that macrophages from VAEC-infected animals showed a 50% reduction in IL-1 activity and a 200% increase in tumour necrosis factor gamma (TNF-γ) activity.

2.2 CASEOUS LYMPHADENITIS

Caseous lymphadenitis is a chronic infectious disease that affects sheep and goats (JOHNSON et al., 1993, MENZIES et al., 2004) and occasionally cattle and humans (McKEAN et al., 2005). Corynebacterium pseudotuberculosis is the aetiological agent of caseous lymphadenitis, from the Actinomyces group, a Gram-positive, short and pleomorphic bacillus (DORELLA et al., 2006), which often appears as an isolated coccoid or in irregular clusters (QUINN et al., 2005). This bacterium is not sporulated, does not have a capsule and is not mobile, although it does have fimbriae. It is a facultative anaerobic bacterium and shows optimum growth at 37 °C, with a pH of 7.0 to 7.2. The colonies are small, whitish and surrounded by a narrow zone of complete haemolysis (QUINN et al., 2005; DORELLA et al., 2006). It is a mesophilic, facultative intracellular bacterium (PRESCOTT et al., 2002; MCKEAN, 2005; MEYER et al., 2005; FONTAINE et al., 2006) that multiplies inside macrophages (CHIRINO-ZÁRRAGA et al., 2006). The virulence of this pathogen is linked to the lipids in its cell wall and the production of an exotoxin, phospholipase D (PLD). In the early stages of infection, phospholipase D can increase the survival and multiplication of this bacterium in the host (QUINN et al., 2005).

The biochemical reactions of Corynebacterium pseudotuberculosis vary considerably, mainly in its ability to ferment. All strains produce acids, but not gas, from some carbon sources, including glucose, fructose, maltose, mannose, sucrose. A reliable test for identifying the bacteria is the API-BioMérieux, (Inc.LaBalme lês Grottes, France), this test consists of 21 biochemical tests and can be carried out in 24-48 h (DORELLA et al., 2006).

The potential of Corynebacterium pseudotuberculosis to survive for many weeks in the environment contributes to its spread in the herd. Transmission between sheep or goats occurs mainly through superficial wounds, which can occur during common procedures such as castration, earring placement, or any generalised injury to the animal's body due to another traumatic event, such as shearing in the case of sheep (DORELLA et al., 2006).

The exact pathogenesis of the infection is poorly understood. It is known that the bacterium has an exotoxin, phospholipase D (COSTA, 2002), considered an important virulence factor that plays a role in the pathogenesis of caseous lymphadenitis (JOHNSON et al., 1993), promoting increased vascular permeability and rupture of small blood vessels at the site of the lesion and consequent extravasation of plasma, facilitating the spread of the bacteria to the lymph nodes (JOHNSON et al., 1993; MCNAMARA et al., 1994; CHAPLIN et al., 1999). In the early stages of infection, this enzyme can increase the survival and multiplication of the bacteria in the host (QUINN et al., 2005). With regard to the biological properties of phospholipase D, it is known to hydrolyse lysophosphatidylcholine and sphingomyelin, essential factors in the formation of abscesses (DERCKSEN et al., 2000; COSTA, 2002).

Another important known virulence factor is the lipids in its cell wall, which are similar to the mycolic acid of Mycobacterium tuberculosis (COSTA, 2002; QUINN et al., 2005); these lipids make it difficult for the bacterium to phagocytose, increasing its virulence factor and promoting toxicity to host cells (TASHJIAN; CAMPBELL, 1983; COSTA, 2002). In addition, Mueller and Pieters (2006) reported various virulence factors and mechanisms of escape from the immune system by mycobacteria, which showed various similarities to C. pseudotuberculosis. In line with this, Tashjian and Campbell (1983) observed that C. pseudotuberculosis is capable of surviving inside phagocytes and can even cause their death, being resistant to death and digestion by macrophages.
Thus, these same bacteria evade the immune system by interrupting the maturation of the phagosome into a phagolysosome and also prevent the development of a localised immune response that can activate macrophages leading to the intraceleular destruction of pathogens (MUELLER; PIETERS, 2006).

It should also be noted that the internalisation of this group of bacteria in macrophages can be mediated by a variety of receptors that lead to their entry and release from the microorganism into the phagosome of the host cell (PIETERS, 2001; RUSSELL, 2001). Once inside the phagosome, the mycobacterium retains or eliminates a series of host molecules, preventing the maturation of the phagosome into a phagolysosome.

A sharp drop in milk, meat and wool production in the case of sheep (ÇETINKAYA et al., 2002; DORELLA et al., 2006), associated with reproductive inefficiency and the death of some adult animals (GATES et al., 1977), are important aspects of losses for producers. The condemnation of carcasses in slaughterhouses and depreciation in the value of leather (due to abscesses caused by the agent) are important economic factors (PATON et al., 1998; NOZAKI et al., 2000), especially for foreign trade (EGGLETON et al., 1991).

Infections by Corynebacterium pseudotuberculosis are highly prevalent in the goat and sheep population in many countries around the world (ELLIS et al., 1991), where there is a large sheep and goat population such as Australia, Argentina, New Zealand, South Africa and countries in the European Community (MOURA COSTA, 2002). Caseous lymphadenitis is one of the most common diseases affecting sheep in Australia. In north-western Australia, the prevalence in flocks is 45 per cent, and the cost of lost production is estimated at 10 to 15 million Australian dollars and 10 million Australian dollars in the food industry (HOGDSON et al., 1994). Çetinkaya et al. (2002) reported that this disease is of great economic importance in goat and sheep flocks in the United States, Canada and Australia, with a reported loss of 17 million dollars per year in Australian production. Canada and Australia report that 21 per cent of animals have caseous lymphadenitis.

In 2003, Carminatti et al. reported that caseous lymphadenitis has a high prevalence in goat herds in the northeast of Brazil, and has also been reported in several Brazilian states.

The spread of infection occurs through pus from ruptured abscesses and oro-nasal discharges between animals with pulmonary infection (CHAPLIN et al., 1999; RIBEIRO et al., 2001; QUINN et al., 2005). Transmission among small ruminants occurs mainly through direct contact with damaged skin or mucous membranes - usually through procedures such as shearing, castration and earring placement - or through damage to the animal's body caused by traumatic events (RIBEIRO et al., 2001; DORELLA et al., 2006). Indirect transmission is also cited in the literature as an important form of contagion and occurs through contamination of the environment, water and food with purulent material from the lymph nodes, which can generate the formation of aerosols (CHAPLIN et al., 1999; RIBEIRO et al., 2001), since the agent can survive in the environment for several months (QUINN et al., 2005). However, Ribeiro et al. (2001) in a study in which, among other objectives, they tried to isolate the bacteria from faeces and the environment (kennel, drinking fountain, feed and facilities) of affected animals, demonstrated the difficulty of isolation, corroborating Radostittis et al. (1994), who refer to this difficulty.

The clinical manifestations of caseous lymphadenitis in small ruminants are mainly characterised by caseous necrosis in the superficial lymph nodes and subcutaneous tissues; in more severe cases it can develop in internal organs such as the lungs, liver, spleen and kidneys - characterising the visceral form of the disease. Abscesses are encapsulated with purulent, dense and caseous material (CHIRINO-ZÁRRAGA et al., 2006, DORELLA et al., 2006; FONTAINE et al., 2006). Affected animals progressively lose weight due to anorexia and can later die from toxemia (CHIRINO-ZÁRRAGA et al., 2006). The disease in humans is similar to that in goats (COSTA,

2002; QUINN et al., 2005).

Diagnosis is based mainly on symptoms (ÇETINKAYA et al., 2002) and on the isolation and identification of the agent from abscess material (QUINN et al., 2005). Serological tests have been used (ÇETINKAYA et al., 2002) and the most commonly used tests are ELISA, complement fixation test, agar gel immunodiffusion test and haemolysis inhibition test (DERCKSEN et al., 2000; RIBEIRO et al., 2001; PRESCOTT et al., 2002). PCR has proved to be a very specific test for inapparent infections (ÇETINKAYA et al., 2002).

The treatment of caseous lymphadenitis is controversial. Some authors, such as Ribeiro et al. (2001) and Senturk and Temizel (2006), advocate the use of antimicrobials, while others, such as Johnson et al. (1993), believe that treatment should not be carried out as it is ineffective because antimicrobials do not reach the lesion in adequate concentrations.

The disease is difficult to eradicate due to its rapid spread when introduced into the herd (ÇETINKAYA et al., 2002). The disease has been controlled by diagnosing and discarding positive animals, with the indirect ELISA test being widely used, making it easier to screen animals (DERCKSEN et al., 2000; CARMINATI et al., 2003; PAULE et al., 2003). The use of vaccines to control caseous lymphadenitis in goats does not show consistent results, as they do not offer adequate immunoprotection to the species (RIBEIRO et al., 1991; FONTAINE et al., 2006).

Because it is a facultative intracellular pathogen, immunity against Corynebacterium pseudotuberculosis is complex and involves a cellular and humoral immune response (ELLIS et al., 1990; PRESCOTT et al., 2002), however, many studies point to a greater cellular response, mainly of the Th1 type, to a humoral response (PEPIN et al., 1997; LAN et al., 1998; SIMMONS et al., 1998). Pepin et al. (1991) observed the relationship between cytokines produced by CD4+ T cells with the development of pyogranulomas and the persistence of the bacteria in the host and described a high production of IFN- γ and low production of IL-4. In contrast, Paule et al. (2003) in a study on the kinetics of IgG and IFN- γ production, showed no correlation between the severity of the infection and the IFN- γ response. In any case, the modulation of the immune response by the control of the expression of MHC class I and II molecules by some cell types, the activation and regulation of phagocyte differentiation and the ability to regulate the activation and differentiation of CD4+ T cells, establish IFN- γ as a key in determining the component and type of function that will be developed during the course of the immune response; thus the role of this cytokine is fundamental in the host's defence against infection by intracellular agents (MEYER et al., 2005).

Pancholi et al. (1993) reported that human monocytes in vitro, chronically infected with *Mycobacterium bovis* bacillus Calmette - Guérin (BCG), had a lower ability to present mycobacterial antigens. Other groups have also demonstrated a reduced ability to process and present antigens as a result of intracellular infection, which can be explained in part by one of the following reasons:

1. Decreased viability of macrophages as a result of infection.
2. Altered ability of macrophages to function properly, for example due to internalisation of the antigen,
3. Change in the expression of surface molecules such as MHC II or other accessory molecules important in T cell stimulation (VANHEYNINGEN et al., 1997).

With regard to the production of immunoglobulins, Desiderio et al. (1979) showed that chronically infected goats had low levels of α2 and β- globulins compared to healthy animals, and these same infected animals had high values for γ- globulin, corroborating Paule et al. (2003) who also observed high levels of IgG. According to Ellis (1988), antibodies against C. pseudotuberculosis exotoxin can protect tissues against exotoxin-mediated damage and the spread of the microorganism and opsonising antibodies can increase neutrophil and macrophage phagocytosis, so the cell-mediated response may be essential for eliminating the microorganism.

2.3 INNATE IMMUNITY

The host's immune response to some invading microorganisms can be divided into innate immunity and adaptive immunity. The adaptive immune response comprises antibody-mediated humoral immunity and T-cell-mediated immunity and usually takes hours or days to initiate. Unlike this, innate immunity triggers a rapid response to invading pathogens and is considered the first line of defence against microorganisms (PLÚDDEMANN et al., 2006).

All healthy individuals are protected by innate immunity, whose characteristics are a limited ability to distinguish one agent from another, and its stereotypical nature, according to which it works in almost the same way against most infectious agents. The components of this immunity include phagocytic cells such as neutrophils, macrophages, dendritic cells and "natural killer" lymphocytes. Of these cells, macrophages deserve special attention as they are targeted by various agents of different species, such as viruses and some bacteria (ABBAS et al., 2000; PENG et al., 2007).

Macrophages are cells derived from blood monocytes, which in turn are derived from cells of the bone marrow haematopoietic system (FELDMAN et al., 2000) and, like macrophages, are cells of the reticuloendothelial system as they have phagocytic characteristics (TIZARD, 1998; FELDMAN et al., 2000; KERR, 2003). In the bone marrow, under the influence of proteins called colony-stimulating factors, monoblasts, which are the precursor cells of monocytes, give rise to promonocytes after mitosis (FELDMAN et al., 2000; KERR, 2003). After two successive mitoses they are released into the bloodstream where they are called monocytes and when they leave the bloodstream they migrate to other tissues and are named after the tissue they migrate to (TIZARD, 1998; FELDMAN et al., 2000). All these cells belong to the mononuclear phagocytic system. This classification involves morphological and functional characteristics, despite all the diversity in different stages of maturation (FELDMAN et al., 2000), 2000), so in the vascular sinusoids of the liver they are called Kupffer cells, in the central nervous system they are called microglial cells, in the bones they are called osteoclasts, in the tissues histiocytes and in the lungs they are classified as alveolar macrophages (TIZARD, 1998; ABBAS et al., 2000; FELDMAN et al., 2000; KERR, 2003; PLÚDDEMANN et al., 2006; GORDON, 2007).

Monocytes are the largest cells among the circulating leucocytes (KERR, 2003; GORDON, 2007). They are characterised by having an elongated nucleus with irregular contours (TIZARD, 1998; KERR, 2003; FELDMAN et al., 2000). The nuclear chromatin may show some areas of condensation. The cytoplasm is made up of a well-developed Golgi complex, some polyribosomes, some granules that vary in size and shape, some vesicles and little rough endoplasmic reticulum cisternae, so they can be mistaken for immature neutrophils (KERR, 2003; FELDMAN et al., 2000).

Morphological, cytochemical and metabolic characteristics depend on the maturity of the monocytes, their place of origin, environmental conditions and degree of stimulation. However, macrophages are generally oval, have elongated or rounded nuclei and prominent nucleoli (TIZARD, 1998). The cytoplasm is abundant with azurophilic granules and vacuoles of varying sizes , mitochondria, rough endoplasmic reticulum and a well-developed Golgi complex (TIZARD, 1998; FELDMAN et al., 2000).

The differentiation of monocytes into macrophages in vitro is accompanied by an increase in cell size, glucose utilisation, lactate production, phagocytic activities, enzyme synthesis and hydrolytic enzyme activity, but a reduction in the ability to produce oxygenated water and superoxide radicals is observed (FELDMAN et al., 2000).

Monocytes and macrophages have surface receptors for the Fc portion of immunoglobulins, as well as receptors for the complement components C3b and C3d. These cells also have receptors for glucocorticoids and hormones such as insulin, glucagon and thyrotropin. These receptors can be altered by in vitro procedures, disease or therapy (FELDMAN et al., 2000; GORDON, 2007).

Complement components such as C3a and C5a are chemotactic for monocytes. One particularity of monocytes is that they are highly chemotactic towards lipids or lipid-rich materials, such as the lipopolysaccharide of Gram-negative bacteria and milk (FELDMAN et al., 2000).

Monocytes fulfil their function after their transformation into macrophages. The phagocytosis capacity of these cells increases as the cells mature from pro-monocytes to macrophages. Monocytes have the ability to phagocytise and remove microorganisms, but to a lesser degree than neutrophils (TIZARD, 1998; FELDMAN et al., 2000; PENG et al., 2007). They are responsible for eliminating intracellular microorganisms (KERR, 2003; FELDMAN et al., 2000), in the face of diseases caused by viruses, they lead to the production of interferon by the cells of the mononuclear phagocytic system and are also responsible for the degradation of antigen-antibody complexes (FELDMAN et al., 2000; PENG et al., 2007).

Some studies in the literature indicate that the C3 receptors present on monocytes are responsible for increasing the adherence of these cells to antigens, but not phagocytosis and oxidative metabolism, a fact that occurs with the Fc receptors, which induce adherence and phagocytosis. However, when the two receptors are combined, they act synergistically (FELDMAN et al., 2000). After phagocytosis, the microorganism interacts with the phagosome and the macrophages synthesise substances that help eliminate the microorganism. These cells perform bactericidal, fungicidal and cytotoxic functions through oxidative metabolism. The products of this metabolism produced by the cells of the mononuclear phagocytic system are smaller than those produced by neutrophils, but sufficient to eliminate the microorganism (FELDMAN et al., 2000).

As well as phagocytosing invading microorganisms, monocytes and macrophages are responsible for removing dead or dying cells (TIZARD, 1998; FELDMAN et al., 2000). Therefore, macrophages recognise changes to the membrane of red blood cells and leukocytes caused by chemical lesions and diseases through opsonisation by antibodies or complement. After phagocytosis, the erythrocyte membrane is digested by enzymes present in the cell vacuoles and the haemoglobin molecules are degraded (FELDMAN et al., 2000).

Macrophages interact with antigens via membrane receptors. Once the antigen has been bound to the macrophages, it is processed and presented to the T and B lymphocytes, triggering the immune response and from this presentation, the lymphocytes produce specific antibodies to the antigens presented by the macrophages (FELDMAN et al., 2000; GORDON, 2007).

When monocytes and macrophages are at rest and receive inflammatory stimuli, they become inflammatory macrophages (TIZARD, 1998). Through the action of substances such as interferons, complement and bacterial products, macrophages become activated (TIZARD, 1998; FELDMAN et al., 2000; PENG et al., 2007) and show many morphological, metabolic and functional changes. They become larger, rich in intracellular organelles such as lysosomes and mitochondria and have a larger Golgi complex. Thus, metabolic activities such as protein synthesis, secretion and synthesis of lysosomal enzymes are increased. In addition, activated macrophages show greater expression of surface receptors and exhibit increased phagocytosis, chemotaxis, digestive, microbicidal and cytotoxic activity (TIZARD, 1998; FELDMAN et al., 2000).

Macrophages are responsible for releasing substances such as lysozyme, complement components and others. When activated, they secrete lysosomal proteases, collagenases, elastases, plasminogen activators and proteins that are essential in regulating immunity such as IL-1, IL-2, IL-12 and TNF-α, which are classified as cytokines (TIZARD, 1998; FELDMAN et al., 2000).

The phagocytosis and intracellular destruction of pathogens by macrophages are important tools of the innate immune system during infection (GORDON, 2007; FRANKENBERG et al., 2008). In this process, pathogens are captured through an extension of the cytoplasmic membrane (pseudopodia) which extends around the ingested particle to form the phagosomal membrane (GORDON, 2007). The phagosomal content resembles the extracellular medium, which is unable to destroy and eliminate the ingested microorganism. However, quickly after the plasma membrane closes, the phagosome undergoes a series of rapid and extensive changes in its composition, which is followed by various fusions and fissions of the membrane and subsequently binds to the lysosome, becoming the phagolysosome (MUELLER; PIETERS, 2006; FRANKENBERG et al., 2008). Phagocytosis is mediated simultaneously and co-operatively by many receptors found on the surface of the macrophage membrane and in intracellular compartments.

An important receptor is the pattern recognition receptor (PRR), which has various functions including opsonisation, activation of complement and the coagulation cascade, phagocytosis, activation of pro-inflammatory signals and induction of apoptosis. Another important component present in macrophages are pathogen-associated molecular patterns (PAMPs), whose ability is to recognise and respond to a vast number of microorganisms. PAMPs act in conjunction with the Toll-like receptor (TLR), which has the ability to recognise distinct PAMPs. TLRs comprise a family of RRP that are capable of recognising different PAMPs. Around 12 TLR families have been identified in mammals, and each member is capable of recognising a distinct PAMP (BANNERMAN et al., 2004).

The phagocytosis of cells of the monocyte-macrophage lineage is dependent not only on the defence structures of these cells, but also on various constituent tools in the structure of microorganisms, which trigger signalling from different receptors that will modulate different responses, often leaving the innate response and moving on to the adaptive response, thus conferring host immunity (UNDERHILL; OZINSKY, 2002). However, some intracellular microorganisms can alter this response by directly interfering with the cell genome, as is the case with some viruses that target cells of the monocyte-macrophage lineage for their replication. In this case, after being phagocytosed, they release their nucleic acid into the cell cytoplasm so that the host cell's DNA, RNA and protein synthesis is inhibited and only the viral genetic information is processed, thus altering cell function and favouring viral replication (TIZARD, 1998).

Intracellular bacteria take advantage of the phagocytosis mechanism to enter the target cells and thus multiply; these microorganisms have some tools to trigger the cellular response and succeed in cell colonisation, as is the case with caseous lymphadenitis, whose virulence factors are capable of causing damage to the host's macrophages, such as cytoplasmic vesiculation, mitochondrial damage and dilation of the endoplasmic reticulum (TASHJIAN et al., 1983). Thus, innate immunity in isolation is effective against many microorganisms, but it can be inefficient when dealing with intracellular pathogens, such as viruses and some bacteria, where the cells of this system, in an attempt to protect the organism, end up serving as a tool for the infection to spread.

CHAPTER 3

OBJECTIVE

To evaluate the effect of VAEC infection on the phagocytic capacity of mononuclear cells for Corynebacterium pseudotuberculosis.

CHAPTER 4

MATERIAL AND METHODS

This chapter will describe the selection of the animals, the sample inclusion criteria for the collections, the analyses to which the samples were subjected and the statistical evaluation.

4.1 ANIMALS EMPLOYED

We used 30 Saanen goats from the experimental herd at the Veterinary Hospital of the Faculty of Veterinary Medicine of the University of São Paulo (FMVZ - USP) and from two goat farms located in the municipality of Ibiúna, in the state of São Paulo.

All the animals were in good nutritional condition with a body score between 3 and 3.5, were not in the puerperal stage and had not been treated with glucocorticoids in the 30 days prior to the experiment.

The animals were divided into two experimental groups according to the results of the immunodiffusion test for anti-VAEC antibodies, with Group 1 consisting of animals serologically negative for CAE and Group 2 of animals serologically positive for CAE.

4.2 BLOOD COLLECTION

A blood sample was collected from each animal by external jugular venipuncture, using a vacuum system and multiple collection needles (25 mm X 8 mm), Vacutainer®[1] , in a siliconised tube without anticoagulant, with a capacity of 10 mL, [1]Becton Dickinson, reference 360212, Plymouth, UK three blood samples in a siliconised tube containing sodium heparin, with a capacity of 10 mL, and one blood sample in a siliconised tube containing tripotassium EDTA at a ratio of 1.5 mg/mL of blood (capacity of 5 mL).

All the samples were identified and sent immediately after collection to the FMVZ - USP Immunodiagnostic Laboratory under refrigeration conditions.

The blood samples from the tubes without anticoagulant were centrifuged for 10 minutes at 1877 x g to obtain serum, from which AEC serodiagnosis was carried out.

The blood samples from the tubes with EDTA were used for the complete blood count and the blood samples from the tubes with heparin were used to recover cells for the phagocytosis tests.

4.3 HAEMATOLOGICAL ANALYSIS

Haematocrit and the total number of erythrocytes and leucocytes were measured as described by Feldman et al. (2000). The differential leucocyte count was carried out using blood smears stained with Rosenfeld's dye (ROSENFELD, 1947) and the leucocyte pattern was differentiated using optical

[1] Becton Dickinson, reference 360212, Plymouth, UK

microscopy at 1000 X magnification.

Table 1 - Reference values for erythrocyte count, mean globular volume and leucogram[1] of healthy goats - São Paulo, 2008

Red blood cells ($x10^6$/ml)	8,0-18,0(13,0)
Globular volume (%)	22,0-38,0 (28,0)
Leucocytes (x 10^3/ml)	4.000- 13.000 (9.000)
Lymphocytes (µl)	2.000-9.000 (5.000)
Neutrophils (µl)	1.200-7.200 (3.250)
Eosinophils (µl)	50-650(450)
Monocytes (µl)	0-550 (250)
Basophils (µl)	0 - 120 (50)

1Values expressed in absolute numbers (Average). Source: Feldman et al., 2000

4.4 SERODIAGNOSIS

The double radial immunodiffusion technique on Ouchterlony agar gel was used to detect serum antibodies to the AEC virus, according to the technique recommended by Cutlip et al. (1977) and recommended by the Office International des Epizooties for screening and international animal transit (OIE, 2007); using the protein antigen (p28) extracted from the AEC virus capsid.

The gel for the IDGA test was prepared following the manufacturer's guidelines[2] for detecting goat arthritis encephalitis virus antibodies. Firstly, the agarose vial supplied in the kit was heated until the agar was fully dissolved and then 14 ml of this solution was poured into 90 mm diameter plastic Petri dishes. The gel was allowed to solidify and the plates were placed under refrigeration to reach a firm consistency so that they could be perforated with a metal mould in the shape of a rosette, containing six outer wells and one central well, all with a diameter of 4 mm and equidistant from the central perforation.

The tests were read in two stages, the first after 48 hours of incubation and the second after 72 hours of incubation. Both were carried out in a dark place with the aid of a torch applied to the underside of the plate to observe the reactions.

4.5 PREPARATION OF BACTERIA FOR IN VITRO TESTING

Corynebacterium pseudotuberculosis was isolated from goats with enlarged lymph nodes by aspiration puncture and subsequently sown on blood agar plates containing 5 % defibrinated sheep's blood, and incubated at 37° C for 72 hours (ÇETINKAYA et al., 2002). identification of the agent was done by staining

Gram tests and biochemical tests were carried out to confirm the agent, using a commercial kit[3] ,

2 CAE Diagnostic Kit (IDGA), Biovetech, Recife - PE.

3 Api Coryne Kit® for Microbiological Diagnosis of Corynebacterium psudotuberculosis, reference 20900, Biomérieux, France.

following the manufacturer's recommendations.

The amount of C. pseudotuberculosis used for the phagocytosis tests was 6 bacteria for each cell (6:1) (RAJAVELU; DAS, 2007; KAPETANOVIC et al., 2007) and was measured using the Mac Farland Scale 10 (tube 10), corresponding to 30 x 10^8 microorganisms/ml (BIER, 1984).

To do this, 0.9% saline solution was used to dilute the bacteria and the concentration was adjusted using a spectrophotometer with a wavelength of 580 nm and transmittance of 4.

4.6 MONOCYTE ISOLATION

Peripheral blood mononuclear cells (PBMC) were isolated by concentration gradient in Ficoll - Plaque Plus®[4] (d = 1.077).

In order to determine whether the sample contained enough cells to carry out the proposed tests and whether these cells had the appropriate vitality (whether they were alive or viable), an aliquot of 10 µL of the cell suspension (cells resuspended in 1mL of RPMI 1640) was added to 90 µL of 0. 1 % Trypan blue solution (MERCK®) and a leucocyte count was carried out in a Neubauer chamber (OLYMPUS microscope),1 % Trypan blue solution (MERCK®) and blood leucocytes were counted in a Neubauer chamber, in the leucocyte quadrant, under light microscopy (OLYMPUS microscope) at 400x magnification.

After viability testing by Trypan blue exclusion, the cells were resuspended in RPMI-1640[5] to reach a final concentration of 1 x 10^7cells/ml.

Inside the wells of polystyrene plates with 24 wells of 16 mm diameter

(COSTAR®)[6] , 13 mm diameter glass coverslips were placed on the plate and 1 ml of the cell suspension was placed on top. The plate was then placed in an oven in 5% CO_2 at 37°C for 1 hour to isolate and adhere the monocytes to the coverslips, according to the technique used by Stabel et al. (1997).

4.7 PHAGOCYTOSIS TEST

After the monocyte incubation period, 20 |il aliquots of the cell suspension, corresponding to 6 x 10^7 bacteria, were added to each well of the plate.

The plates were incubated at 37°C for 2 hours in 5% CO_2, and fixed with 0.5% glutaraldehyde for 10 minutes.

Initially, the coverslips were read using optical microscopy at 1000 X magnification, after staining with Rosenfeld's dye at a 1:2 dilution, i.e. 1 mL of dye and 2 mL of distilled water for 4

[4] Ficoll -Plaque Plus GE Healthcare, reference 17-1440-03, d= 1.077, Uppsala, Sweden.
[5] RPMI 1640 Sigma Aldrich, reference R7638, Saint Louis, USA
[6] Corning Incorporated COSTAR, reference 3524, Corning, USA

minutes, where 400 cells were counted. To categorise and quantify the monocyte-macrophage series, the cells were classified into six groups:

1. Adhered monocytes
2. Monocytes phagocytising Corynebacterium pseudotuberculosis
3. Adhered macrophages
4. Spreading macrophages
5. Macrophages that phagocytised up to 12 Corynebacterium pseudotuberculosis (Phagocytosis +).
6. Macrophages that phagocytised more than 12 Corynebacterium pseudotuberculosis (Phagocytosis ++)

4.8 CHARACTERISATION OF CELL GROUPS

In order to carry out this study, it was essential to differentiate and discriminate between the different cell groups according to their morphofunctional characteristics, as described below:

4.8.1 Adhered Monocytes

Cells with scarce cytoplasm were characterised as monocytes, although the nucleus was considered pleomorphic, with a predominance of reniform and oval shapes (Figure 7).

4.8.2 Monocytes phagocytising Corynebacterium pseudotuberculosis

Monocytes with bacterial particles inside small cytoplasmic vacuoles, indicating phagocytosis (Figure 10).

4.8.3 Adhered Macrophages

Macrophages had in common an abundant cytoplasm, with the presence of small vacuoles, and variations in size were often found. The nucleus usually had a reniform or rounded shape and was peripherally or centrally located (Figure 8).

4.8.4 Sprawling macrophages

Similar characteristics to the previous one, but the presence of cytoplasmic projections and vacuoles was observed (Figure 9).

4.8.5 Phagocytosis +

Macrophages that showed particles (up to twelve bacteria) inside cytoplasmic vacuoles indicated phagocytosis (Figure 11).

4.8.6 Phagocytosis ++

Macrophages that showed particles (more than twelve bacteria) inside cytoplasmic vacuoles indicated phagocytosis (Figure 12).

4.9 STATISTICAL ANALYSIS

The normality of the distribution of the observed results was checked using the Anderson-Darling test and their homoscedasticity using the F test. The variance analysis test (One-way ANOVA) was used to assess the differences between the means of the results.

To assess the correlations between the observed data, Pearson's correlation coefficient was analysed, using the classification criteria indicated by Callegari-Jacques (2003).

For all the results, analyses with $p<0.05$ were considered significant. Data is expressed as mean (±standard deviation).

Statistical evaluations used MINITAB® statistical software, version 15 (Global Tech Informática™, Belo Horizonte, MG).

CHAPTER 5

RESULTS

The presence of VAEC seropositive animals was verified in the populations studied. These results led to the random selection of goats to make up the experimental groups, from which blood samples were obtained and submitted for evaluation of the spreading and phagocytic capacity of the cells of the monocyte-macrophage series in vitro against the bacterium Corynebacterium pseudotuberculosis.

5.1 SCREENING AND FORMATION OF EXPERIMENTAL GROUPS

Eighty adult animals were screened from the experimental herd at the Veterinary Hospital of the Faculty of Veterinary Medicine of the University of São Paulo (FMVZ - USP) and from two goats located in the municipality of Ibiúna (São Paulo).

According to the results obtained using the IDAG technique to check for serum antibodies to the AEC virus, 48.75 per cent of the animals were seropositive and 51.25 per cent seronegative (Figure 1), corresponding to 39 and 41 animals respectively.

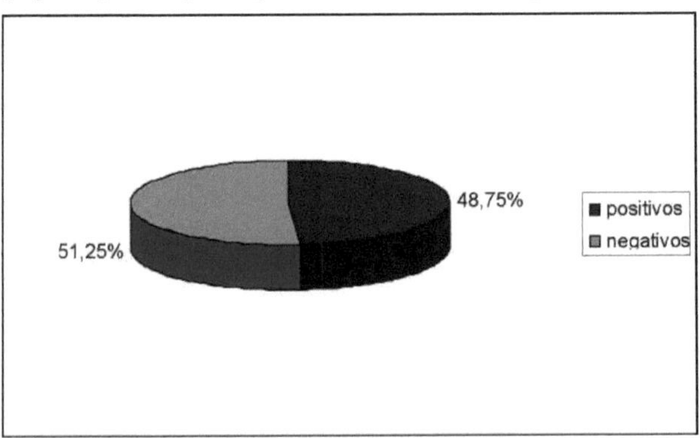

Figure 1- Distribution of agar gel immunodiffusion (AGID) results for the diagnosis of caprine encephalitis arthritis in 80 Saanen goats - São Paulo - 2008

To make up the experimental group, 30 animals were selected and allocated to two different groups: one group was made up of 15 animals that were negative to the serological test for detecting serum antibodies to the AEC virus and the other group was made up of 15 animals that were reactive to the test, thus being called the positive group.

5.2 EVALUATION OF THE BLOOD COUNT OF THE SELECTED ANIMALS

The results of the haematocrit, total erythrocyte and leukocyte count, as well as the absolute differential leukocyte count of the selected animals are broken down according to serodiagnosis, shown in Table 1 and Figures 2, 3, 4 and 5.

Table 1- Average results of erythrocyte and leucocyte counts and percentage of average globular volume, in absolute numbers (mean + standard deviation) and %, respectively, of 30 Saanen animals, separated according to experimental group - São Paulo - 2008

	Negative Group (n = 15)	Positive Group (n = 18)	
Parameters	Mean (+ SD)	Mean (+ SD)	p
Red blood cells (x 10^6 /ml)	13,89 (+ 3,36)	13,92 (+ 2,44)	0,97
Haematocrit (%)	28,53 (+ 6,09)	26,40 (+ 5,22)	0,31
Leucocytes (x 10^3/ml)	15,05 (+ 4,26)	13,78 (+ 2,05)	0,30
Lymphocytes (µl)	8,17 (+ 3,98)	6,59 (+ 2,63)	0,21
Neutrophils (µl)	6,43 (+ 2,12)	6,72 (+ 1,96)	0,70
Eosinophils (µl)	0,20 (+ 0,18)	0,32(+ 0,33)	0,24
Monocytes (µl)	0,25 (+ 0,23)	0,15 (+ 0,07)	0,11
Basophils (µl)	0,00	0,00	

SD = Standard Deviation

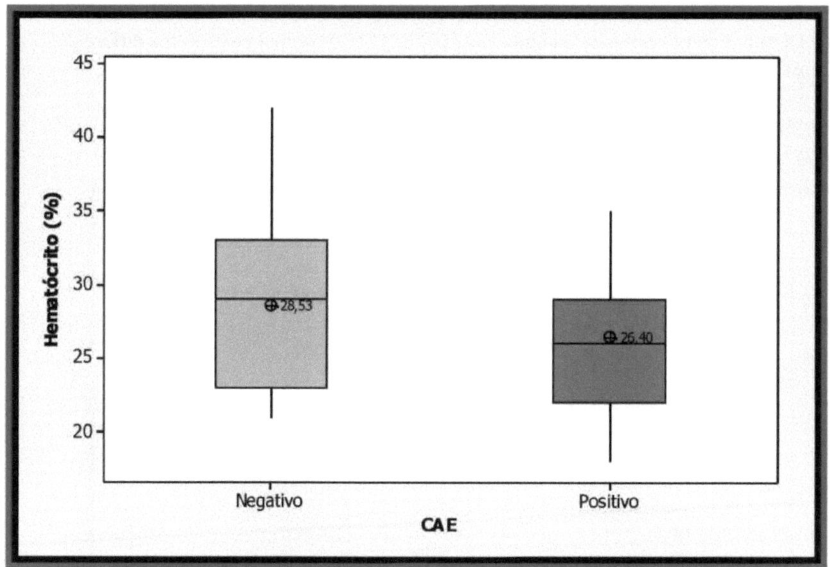

Figura 2 - Distribution of globular volume data (%) of 30 Saanen goats in the different experimental groups - São Paulo - 2008

The average globular volume of the animals in the experimental groups showed no statistical difference (Table 1 and Figure 2) and made it possible to rule out dehydration and anaemia.

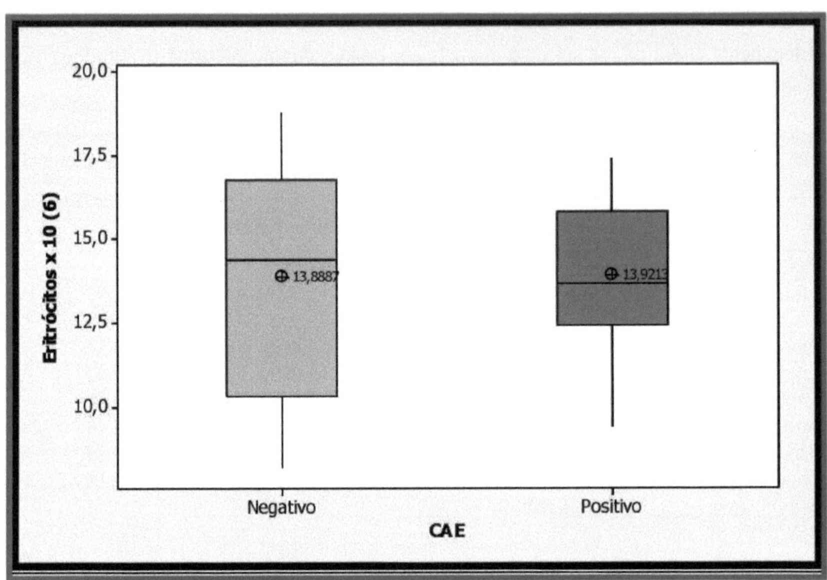

Figura 3 - Distribution of erythrocyte count data (10^6/ml) of 30 Saanen goats in the different experimental groups - São Paulo - 2008

The erythrocyte count showed no difference between the animals in the groups (Table 1 and Figure 3) and made it possible to rule out anaemia.

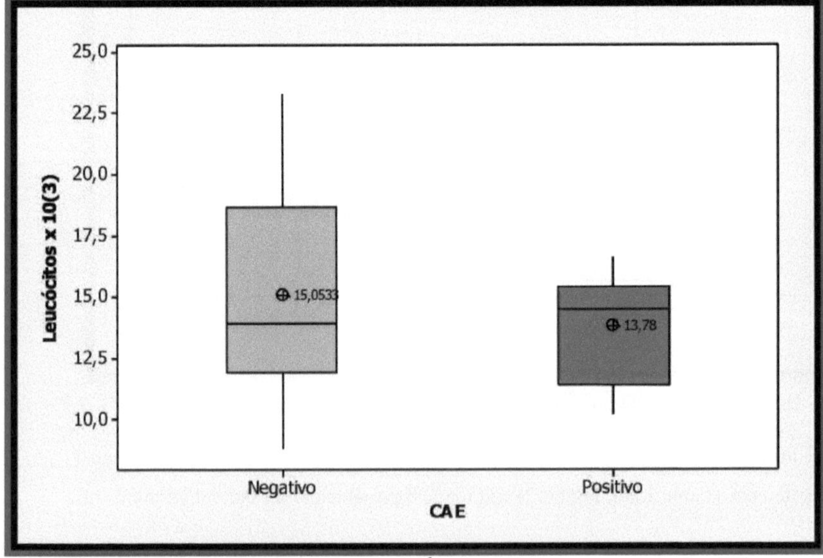

Figura 4 - Distribution of leucocyte counts (10^3/ml) of 30 Saanen goats in the different experimental groups - São Paulo - 2008

As shown in Table 1 and Figure 4, the leucocyte values did not differ between the groups, confirming the homogeneity in the formation of the experimental groups. The same was true of the absolute and relative counts of each leukocyte population (Table 2 and Figures 5 and 6), where the animals in the different groups analysed showed uniformity.

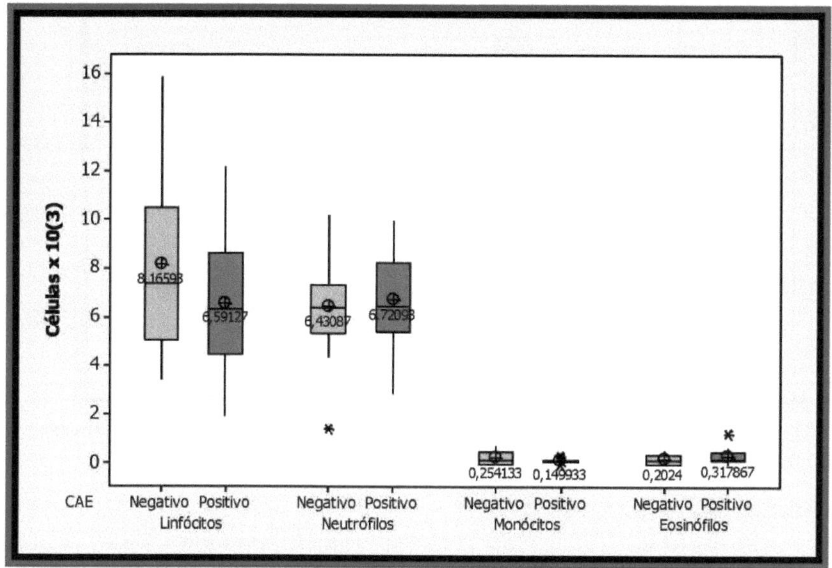

Figura 5 - Distribution of the absolute count data of the different leucocyte populations (10^3/ml) of the 30 Saanen goats in the different experimental groups - São Paulo - 2008

Table 2 - Mean results and standard deviations of the relative differential count of blood leucocytes (%) (mean + standard deviation), of goats distributed according to experimental group - São Paulo - 2008

	Negative Group (n = 15)	Positive Group (n = 18)	
Parameters (%)	Mean (+ SD)	Mean (+ SD)	p
Lymphocytes	52,47 (+ 15,21)	47,00 (+ 15,29)	0,33
Neutrophils	44,33 (+ 15,27)	49,53 (+ 14,96)	0,35
Eosinophils	1,53 (+ 1,40)	2,40 (+ 2,35)	0,23
Monocytes	1,66 (+ 1,67)	1,07 (+ 0,46)	0,19
Basophils	0,00	0,00	

SD = Standard Deviation

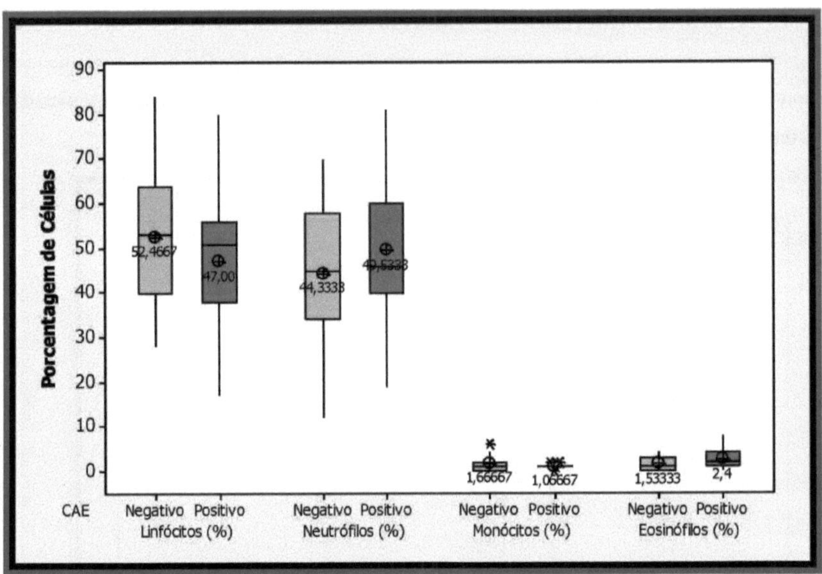

Figure 6 - Distribution of the results of the relative count of the different leucocyte populations (10^3/ml) of the 30 Saanen goats in the different experimental groups - São Paulo - 2008

5.3 SPREADING AND PHAGOCYTOSIS TEST

The evaluation of the spreading and phagocytic capacity of the cells of the monocyte-macrophage series of the animals in the experimental groups against the bacterium Corynecbacterium pseudotuberculosis showed no significant difference (Table 3).

Table 3 - Evaluation of in vitro phagocytosis (%) of Corynebacterium pseudotuberculosis by cells of the monocyte-macrophage series obtained from blood samples (mean + standard deviation) of goats negative for VAEC serodiagnosis - São Paulo - 2008

	Negative (n= 15)	Positive (n= 18)	p
Monocyte	9,03 (3,67)	11,51 (4,14)	0,09
Macrophage	28,49 (8,83)	23,49 (9,93)	0,18
Spreading Macrophage	10,03 (3,63)	9,21 (3,76	0,55
Total phagocytosis	52,39 (8,93)	55,45 (11,12)	0,41

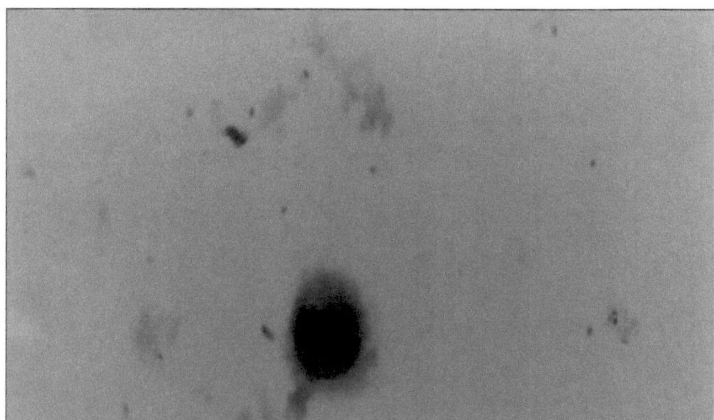

Figure 07 - Photo micrograph of adhered goat monocyte with scarce cytoplasm and abundant nucleus

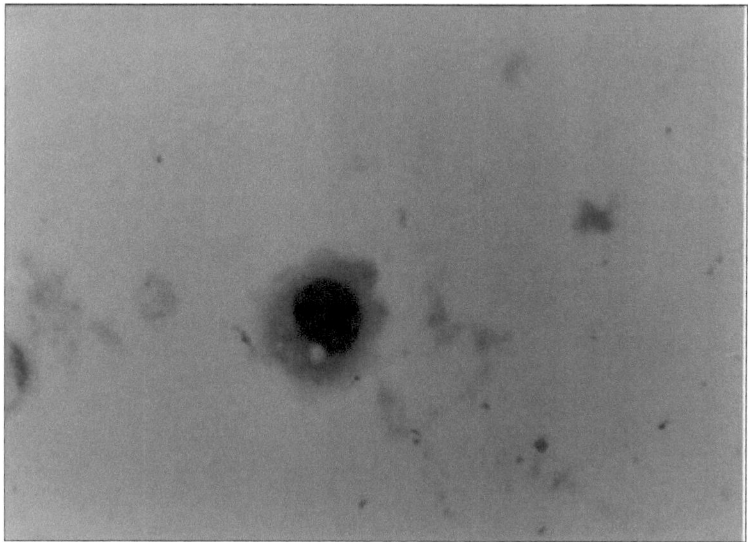

Figura 8 - Photo micrograph of an adhered goat macrophage with abundant cytoplasm and the presence of cytoplasmic vacuoles and a nucleus with loose chromatin

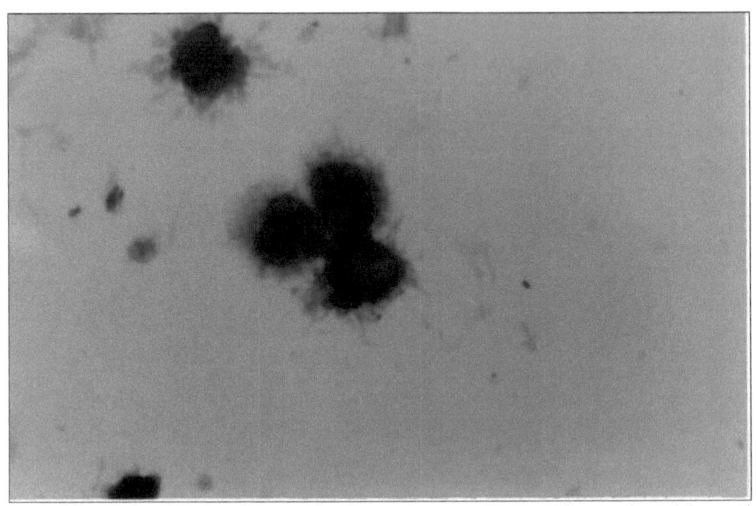

Figura 9 - Photo micrograph of a goat macrophage with pseudopod formation.

However, when macrophage phagocytosis was broken down according to the number of phagocytosed particles (Corynebacteium pseudotuberculosis), a significant difference was observed between the groups formed according to the AEC serodiagnosis result, as shown in Table 4.

Table 4 - Evaluation of in vitro phagocytosis rates (%) broken down into two different groups according to the number of phagocytosed particles (Corynebacterium pseudotuberculosis) by cells of the monocyte-macrophage series (mean + standard deviation) of Saanen goats, separated according to serodiagnosis for AEC - São Paulo - 2008

	Negative (n= 15)	Positive (n= 15)	p
Monocyte phagocytosis	2,081 (1,55)	2,89 (2,19)	0,250
Phagocytosis +	34,87 (5,91)	27,67 (4,83)	0,012
Phagocytosis ++	15,45 (8,62)	24,88 (10,44)	0,001

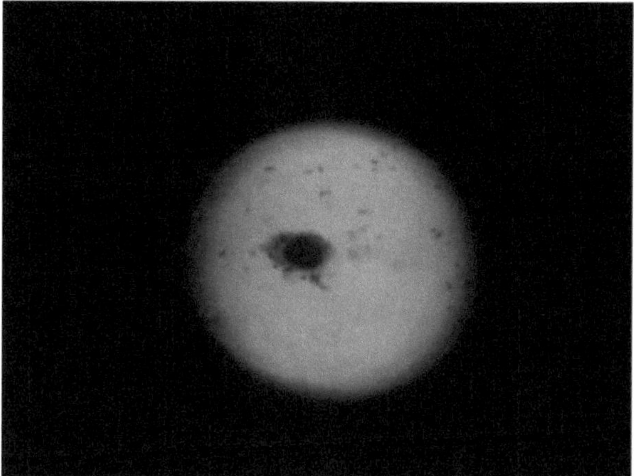

Figura 10 - Photo micrograph of goat monocytes phagocytising the bacterium Corynebacterium pseudotuberculosis

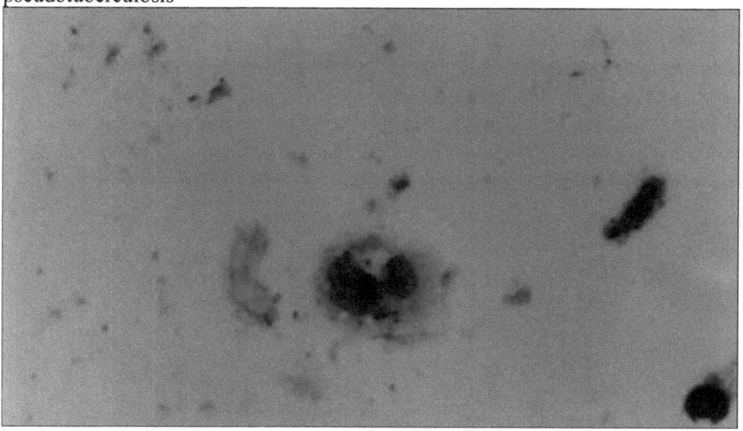

Figura 11 - Photo micrograph of a goat macrophage phagocytising (+) the bacterium Corynebacterium pseudotuberculosis

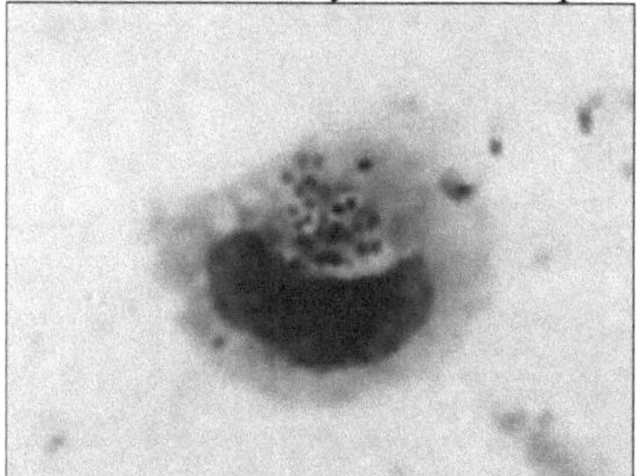

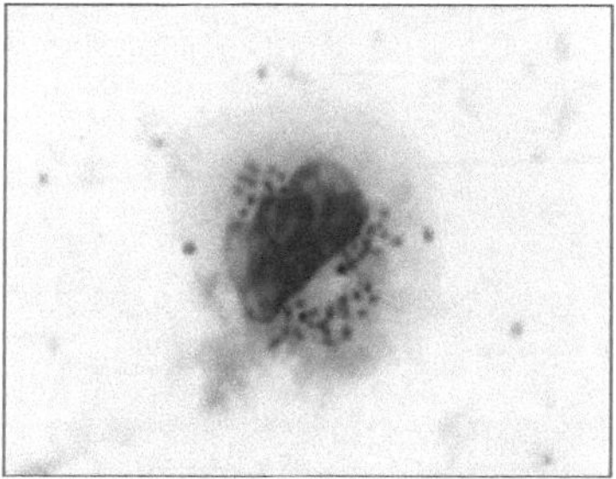

Figura 12 - Photo micrograph of a phagocytosing goat macrophage (++), showing abundant and vacuolised cytoplasm containing in some of them the bacterium Corynebacterium pseudotuberculosis

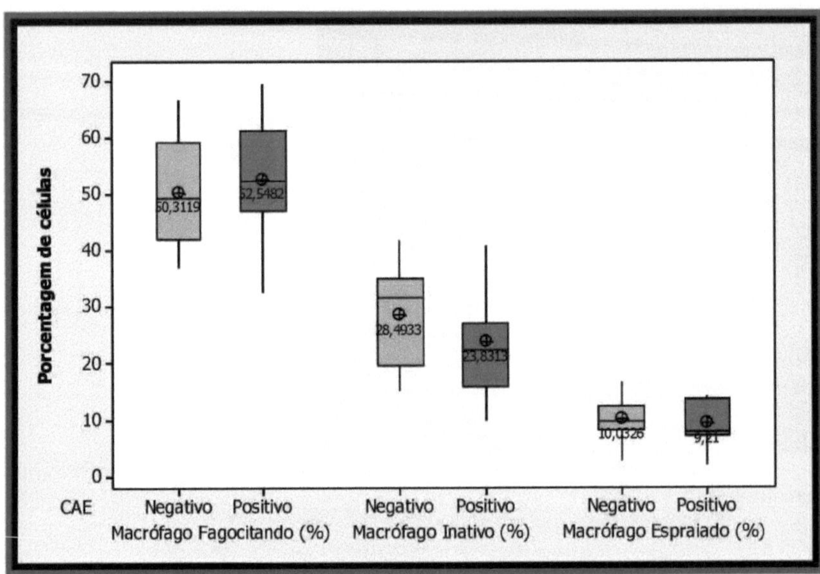

Figura 13 - Distribution of data on the different percentages of macrophages, macrophages that spread and macrophages that phagocytised Corynebacterium pseudotuberculosis in the 30 Saanen goats in the different experimental groups - São Paulo - 2008

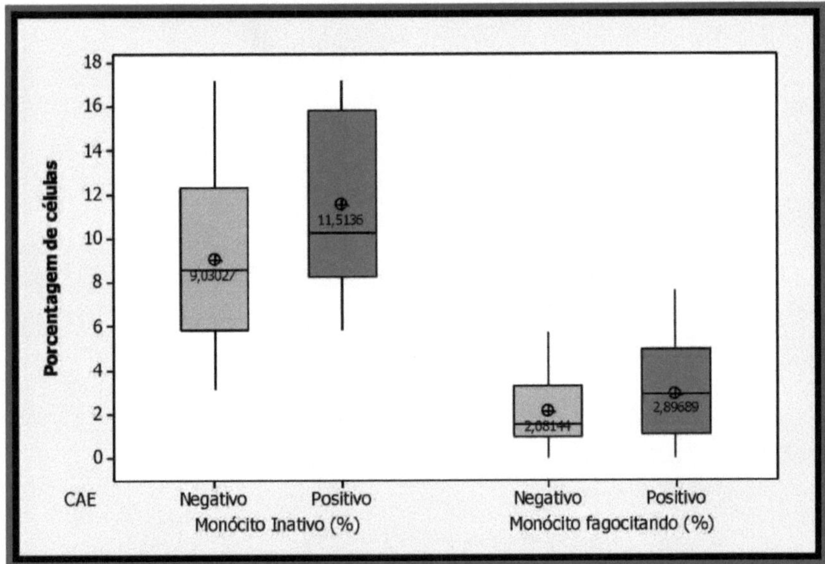

Figura 14 - Distribution of data on the different percentages of monocytes and monocytes that phagocytised Corynebacterium pseudotuberculosis in the 30 Saanen goats in the different experimental groups - São Paulo - 2008

As illustrated in figure 15 and table 4, there was no significant difference in the phagocytic capacity of monocytes between the groups. However, there was a quantitative difference in phagocytosis between the macrophages, i.e. the macrophages in the positive group had a higher percentage of cells phagocytising more particles (above 12 bacteria) ($p<0.001$), as shown in Figures 12 and 15, compared to the group of negative animals which had macrophages phagocytising up to 12 bacteria ($p<0.012$) (Figure 11).

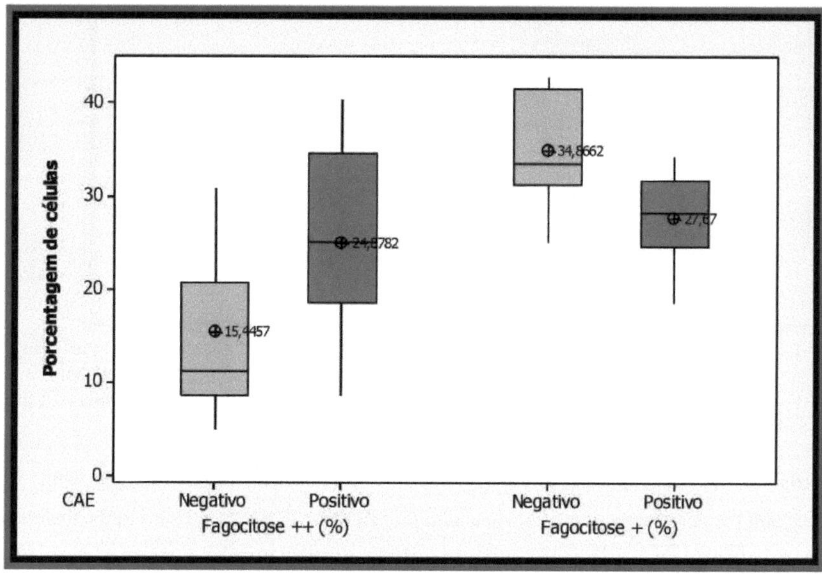

Figura 15 - Distribution of data on the different percentages of macrophages that phagocytised up to 12 Corynebacterium pseudotuberculosis (Phagocytosis +) and macrophages that phagocytised more than 12 Corynebacterium pseudotuberculosis (Phagocytosis ++) in the 30 Saanen goats in the different experimental groups - São Paulo - 2008

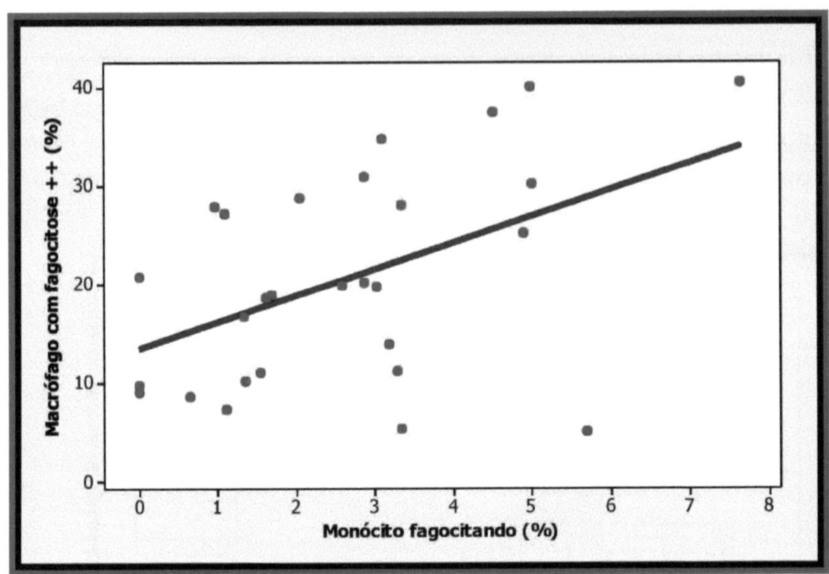

Figure 16 - Correlation between the percentage of monocytes that phagocytosed up to 12 particles (Corynebacterium pseudotuberculosis) (Phagocytosis +) and macrophages that phagocytosed more than 12 bacteria (Phagocytosis ++) of the 30 Saanen goats in the different experimental groups - São Paulo - 2008

There was a positive correlation between the percentage of macrophages with ++ phagocytosis and the percentage of phagocytosing monocytes (r = 0.488; p = 0.006) in the different groups (Figures 10 and 16).

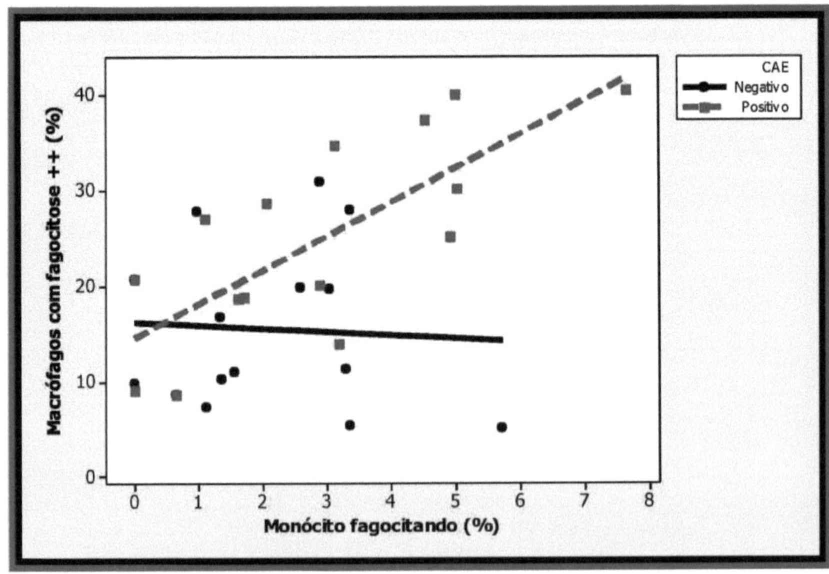

Figure 17 - Correlation between the percentage of monocytes that phagocytosed up to 12 particles (Corynebacterium pseudotuberculosis) (Phagocytosis +) and macrophages that phagocytosed more than 12 bacteria (Phagocytosis ++) of the 30 Saanen goats in the different experimental groups - São Paulo - 2008

Furthermore, there was a significant correlation ($r = 0.748$, $p < 0.001$) between the percentage of macrophages with ++ phagocytosis and the percentage of phagocytosing monocytes (Figure 17) in the seropositive animals, which was not found in the group of seronegative animals ($p < 0.49$).

CHAPTER 6

DISCUSSION

Caprine encephalitis virus arthritis and caseous lymphadenitis are two important chronic diseases that affect goats and are caused by a lentivirus and the bacterium Corynebacterium pseudotuberculosis, respectively. The interaction between the aetiological agents and the host's immune response has been the subject of many studies, but this relationship has not been fully elucidated. Furthermore, the two diseases are studied in isolation, as well as the interaction between bacteria and viruses. Thus, assuming that the two diseases have causal agents from different species, but that they share a common tropism for the same cell (LARA et al., 2005; CHIRINO- ZÁRRAGA et al., 2006) and that studies on the two diseases are usually carried out in isolation, the aim of this study was to assess the in vitro phagocytic function of monocyte-macrophage cells from VAEC-infected animals using the bacterium Corynebacterium pseudotuberculosis as an antigenic challenge, based on the hypothesis that these cells from animals carrying the virus have compromised or altered phagocytic function, predisposing carriers to future infections, including caseous lymphadenitis.

The VAEC screening of animals from three different locations showed that 48.75% of the animals screened were carriers of the virus. This result was not intended to validate the finding epidemiologically, but it did show that the disease is common in herds and was in line with the rates quoted in the literature, which state that this is a disease found worldwide in herds with high rates of infected animals, regardless of breed, sex and age, with dairy herds showing the highest prevalence of the disease (CUTLIP et al., 1992; BELANGER; LEBOEUF, 1993; PINHEIRO et al., 2001; TORRES-ACOSTA et al., 2003, AL-QUDAH et al., 2006; GUFLER et al., 2007).

The test chosen to identify animals affected by the AEC virus in this study was agar gel immunodiffusion, the most widely used test to detect anti-VAEC antibodies (LARA et al., 2003; CORTEZ-MOREIRA et al., 2005). This technique is recommended by the Office International des Epizooties (OIE) for screening and transit of animals, and by the International Animal Health Code for importing and exporting animals, and has 100 per cent specificity (ANDRÉS et al., 2005; CORTEZ-MOREIRA et al., 2005). However, the sensitivity of this test is controversial, as there are reports in the literature of 70 to 91 per cent (ANDRÉS et al., 2005, BRINKHOF; VAN MAANEN, 2007).

Comparing the sensitivity of the IDGA to the ELISA test, the latter has shown greater sensitivity than the former, especially in cases of animals with late seroconversion. However, due to its specificity, the IDGA does not point to false-positive results like the ELISA test (ANDRÉS et al., 2005; CORTEZ-MOREIRA et al., 2005; BRINKHOF; VAN MAANEN, 2007).

A comparative study between the PCR and IDGA tests showed that the former does not have the specificity of the latter, and suggested using it as an auxiliary tool to IDGA, since the result showed that PCR detected a smaller number of positive animals, but a larger number of negative animals (RUTKOSKI et al., 2001).

As this study sought to assess the interrelationship between two important diseases that affect goats, we tried to exclude the possibility of other disorders by assessing the erythrocyte and leucocyte series. Thus, the globular volume of seropositive animals when compared to seronegative animals did not differ from each other, and was also within pre-established standards for goats (FELDMAN et al., 2000). Similarly, the erythrocyte count between the animals in the different groups was within normal range when the results were compared with the normal reference values cited in the literature (FELDMAN et al., 2000; VIANA, 2001).

The leucocyte count showed no significant difference between the groups, but the values were higher than those proposed by Feldman et al. (2000). When comparing the results with the Brazilian reference values recommended by Viana (2001), who analysed the different stages of pregnancy and puerperium on the blood count of Saanen goats raised in the state of São Paulo, the absolute and relative counts of the different leucocyte populations were within the range for healthy goats. These data may represent a panorama that is closer to the Brazilian reality, but may differ in some aspects from international parameters due to the different antigenic challenges that our animals are subjected to and the different health and production management conditions.

Once the sample inclusion criteria for this study had been established, we went on to consider the characteristics of the techniques chosen to assess phagocytic function specifically related to Corynebacterium pseudotuberculosis.

The amount of bacteria needed to induce phagocytosis differed from the ratio (10:1 - bacteria cells) used by most researchers (KAPETANOVIC et al., 2007, RAJAVELU; DAS, 2007; WEISS et al., 2008). However, other studies have used a lower bacterial concentration per phagocyte, especially when considering studies that have used Corynebacterium pseudotuberculosis or other actinomycetes in a ratio ranging from 1 to 5 bacteria per cell (TASHJIAN; CAMPBELL, 1983; GOLLNICK et al., 2007; JORDAO et al., 2008).

At the beginning of this study, we tried to work with a 10:1 ratio, but we noticed a large amount of cell debris. By reducing this ratio and working with a ratio of six bacteria to one mononuclear cell, a large number of intact phagocytes were observed at various stages of maturation, i.e. from monocytes to highly reactive macrophages. This difference in quantity can be explained by the fact that the other authors worked with other animal and bacterial species.

The monocyte-macrophage cell adherence technique used in this study proved to be efficient for this purpose, but lymphocyte adherence was also observed. This data is divergent in the literature, as Stabel et al. (1997) studied the function of bovine peripheral blood monocytes, but did not describe the adherence of lymphocytes. However, Goddeeris et al. (1986), in a comparative study of different techniques for adhering bovine monocytes, described that the technique for separating mononuclear cells by adhering them to polystyrene plates resulted in only 60% of monocytes.

The time used for adhesion and phagocytosis of the bacteria made it possible to observe various stages of cell maturation. This shows that the bacteria as an antigenic challenge, as well as the amount used per cell and the incubation time, were able to induce an immune response from the phagocytes. Furthermore, it was observed that there was no cell death during the incubation period used, corroborating Tashjian and Campbell (1983) who observed that C. pseudotuberculosis is capable of surviving inside phagocytes and can cause them to die. Furthermore, the destruction of macrophages was first evident in the samples between 1 and 4 hours, but generalised damage was not observed until 8 hours had elapsed. Cell destruction was evidenced by the large amount of debris in the material examined, which may be due to the action of the phospholipase D endotoxin produced by C. pseudotuberculosis. This bacterium is resistant to death and digestion by macrophages and this resistance is probably due to the presence of a lipid layer in the bacterial wall, which is also an important virulence factor.

Based on the stage and presence of phagocytosis, we tried to classify the cells as follows: adhered monocytes, monocytes phagocytosing C. pseudotuberculosis, adhered macrophages, spreading macrophages and phagocytosing macrophages. An unexpected finding, but one that was observed in this study, was the presence of two distinct classes of phagocytosis by macrophages classified as + and ++. To determine this classification, the number of particles inside the cell vacuoles was taken into account and it was observed that the cells that ingested a smaller number of bacteria had up to twelve particles and were therefore considered to have + phagocytosis. The others generally phagocytosed a countless number of bacteria engulfed in phagolysosomes and were classified as phagocytosis ++. Thus, the division of phagocytosis into different scores according to the number of particles was fundamental in order to verify the difference between the phagocytic capacity of the different groups. Heterogeneity in cellular phagocytic capacity has already been described in other studies, and it has also been suggested that simply quantifying phagocytes without evaluating the number of particles phagocytosed would be of limited relevance (RIVAS et al., 2002). Therefore, the phagocytosis group was implemented by phagocytosis status, thus becoming phagocytosis + (Figure 11) and phagocytosis ++ (Figure 12).

Analysing the experimental groups revealed three important phenomena: firstly, there was a higher percentage of macrophages with ++ phagocytosis in the cells obtained from the group of animals that tested positive for serum AEC virus antibodies when compared to the cells from the group of animals that tested negative for serology ($p = 0.001$) (Table 4 and Figure 15).

Secondly, there was a higher percentage of macrophages with phagocytosis + in the cells obtained from the group of seronegative animals, when compared to the cells obtained from the group of seropositive animals ($p = 0.012$) (Table 4 and Figure 15).

Thirdly, there was a positive correlation in the group of positive animals between phagocytosing ++ macrophages and phagocytosing monocytes ($r = 0.488$, $p = 0.006$) (Figures 16 and 17). This relationship suggests a greater phagocytic capacity of the monocyte-macrophage series, regardless of their state of maturation, but other authors have reported that monocyte-derived macrophages are similar to monocytes, although they exhibit a greater phagocytic capacity, and that the maturation of monocytes into macrophages may increase the expression of CR4, which contributes to phagocytosis (MYONES et al., 1988; WOO et al., 2006). In addition, it is also proposed that the lower infection of monocytes by VAEC can be explained in part by the lower number of receptors for the virus or even their absence (GENDELMAN et al., 1986). It has also been reported that VAEC can alter the responsiveness of cytokine production by monocytes (WERLING et al., 1994) and that it can alter the ability of these cells to act synergistically with lymphocytes in inducing the immune response. This suggests that other mechanisms may be involved in regulating the phagocytic response of these cells in VAEC-infected animals.

However, the total percentage of phagocytosing macrophages (phagocytosis ++ and phagocytosis +), as well as the total percentage of phagocytosing cells (macrophages and monocytes) did not differ between the groups, as has been reported in the literature (ANDERSON et al., 1983). This is an important piece of data, which shows that there is no difference in the number of cells carrying out phagocytosis, regardless of whether the animal has anti-VAEC antibodies or not. However, the phagocytic capacity varied, with cells derived from seropositive animals showing a greater capacity for phagocytosis when compared to cells from negative animals.

Mononuclear phagocytes play a fundamental role in the pathogenesis of C. pseudotuberculosis infection, providing an intracellular niche for the survival and multiplication of this coco-bacillus. It is a facultative intracellular agent, which is rapidly phagocytosed by macrophages; however, even with the formation of the phagolysosome, the bacterium continues to multiply, leading to cell death and release of the bacterium and subsequently causing a necrotic lesion (WALKER et al., 1994). The ability of C. pseudotuberculosis to survive and proliferate within macrophages is also a form of dissemination through the lymphatic system (BILLINGTON et al., 2002). It should also be considered that the lymph node is an important reservoir for VAEC replication (RAVAZZOLO et al., 2006) and also an important multiplication site for Corynebacterium pseudotuberculosis, since once infected, the macrophages move on to the lymph nodes that drain the region from the initial lesion (KURIA et al., 2001). Viral transcription has also been seen in non-inflamed tissues in smaller numbers than in inflamed tissues (ZINK et al., 1990). Thus, viral replication is also reported to be greater in macrophages than in monocytes (ANDERSON;

ANDERSON, 1982; ANDERSON et al., 1983; ZINK; NARAYAN, 1989).

When checking the pathogenicity of other actinomycetes that are very similar to Corynebacterium pseudotuberculosis, similarities were observed in the mechanism of escape from the immune system. These similarities between this bacterial group are reinforced by the presence of cell wall antigens that these agents have in common, which can also cause false-positive results in the tuberculin test in animals infected with C. pseudotuberculosis (WILLIAMSON, 2001).

In addition, these same bacteria evade the immune system by interrupting the maturation of the phagosome into a phagolysosome and also prevent the development of a localised immune response that can activate macrophages leading to the intracellular destruction of pathogens (MUELLER; PIETERS, 2006).

In addition, the entry of this group of bacteria into phagocytic cells can be mediated by a variety of receptors that lead to their entry and release of the microorganism into the phagosome of the host cell (PIETERS, 2001;,RUSSELL, 2001). Within the phagosome, the mycobacteria retain or eliminate a series of molecules from the host, leading to the prevention of the maturation of the phagosome into a phagolysosome. However, the mechanisms used by the bacteria to modulate and block the maturation of phagosomes have not been fully elucidated. However, evidence suggests that certain signalling events that normally accompany phagosome maturation are inhibited or modulated by these intracellular bacteria (PIETERS; MUELLER, 2006). For example, Mycobacterium tuberculosis secretes a lipid phosphatase that cleaves PI3P (Phosphatidylinositol 3-phosphate) and blocks the fusion of the phagosome to the endosome in in vitro assays, thus contributing to the inhibition of phagosome maturation (VERGNE et al., 2005).

Mycobacteria are able to block the activation of T cells by macrophages which may be correlated with the bacillus' ability to induce the production of cytokines such as IL-1, IL-6 and FNT-α at inhibitory levels within granulomas (VAN HEYNINIGEN et al., 1987). However, this occurs even if intracellular mycobacteria minimise the ability of macrophages to induce a localised cellular immune response. The evasion of this delayed immune response may be, at least in part, due to the ability of mycobacteria to produce anergic infection of macrophages by activating cytokines such as IFN- γ that may be the result of bacterial components that are expressed within the infected cell (TING et al., 1999). Weiss et al. (2004) provided evidence of increased IL-10 expression in macrophages derived from monocytes infected with M. tuberculosis and that the neutralisation of IL-10 enabled the digestion of M. tuberculosis.

From the above, the results of this study point to a suggestion of greater dissemination of lymphadenitis, as the greater quantity of phagocytosed bacterial particles in VAEC-infected animals could facilitate the dissemination of the bacteria to other tissues and the formation of new granulomas. However, many studies have evaluated the survival of C. pseudotuberculosis within macrophages, but it should be considered that the extracellular phase of infection by C. pseudotuberculosis may be important in the transmission of this bacterium between cells, in particular the involvement of the host response to this phase of infection should also be considered.

In line with this, it has been reported that the pulmonary form of *Corynebacterium pseudotuberculosis* infection occurs more frequently in sheep infected with lentiviruses (GATES et al., 1977; BRODIE et al., 1992). It has also been reported in humans that *Mycobacterium tuberculosis* infection is more common in individuals with the human immunodeficiency virus (HIV) and that this bacterial disease can accelerate the progression of the latter (ELLNER, 1990). These two infections appear to have a synergistic effect, causing a shift in favour of their etiological agents that cannot be reversed by treatment with antimycobacterial agents (WALLIS; ELLNER, 1994). It was then suggested that mycobacterial infections could cause an increase in the production of IL-6, which suppresses cell-mediated immunity. Thus, IL-6 as well as IL-1 and FNT-α have been implicated in the induction of HIV replication (VANHEYNINGEN et al., 1997). Thus, since VAEC belongs to the same family and genus as HIV (QUINN et al., 2005) and *C. pseudotuberculosis* is an actinomycete like *Mycobacterium tuberculosis* (DORELLA et al., 2006), and their similarities in modulating the immune response, it is believed that the progression of these diseases may also have a synergistic effect on each other. Studies have also shown that soluble mediators secreted in the response to this bacterium can modulate the replication of lentiviruses, and by extension favour the progression of the disease in sheep infected with both diseases (ELLIS et al., 1994). Although soluble mediators were not analysed in this study, there was a clear difference in the intensity of phagocytosis in the animals with AEC, pointing to the same reasoning.

CHAPTER 7

CONCLUSION

This study led to the conclusion that caprine encephalitis virus arthritis interferes with the innate immunity of virus-infected animals, since an increase in the intensity of macrophage phagocytosis and an increase in the number of phagocytosing monocytes were observed in the positive group, suggesting that AEC predisposes animals to caseous lymphadenitis.

REFERENCES

ADAMS, D. S.; KLEVJER-ANDERSON, P.; CARLSON, J. L.; MCGUIRE, T. C.; GORHAM, J. R. Transmission and control of caprine arthritis-encephalitis virus. American Journal of Veterinary Research, v. 44, n. 9, p. 1670-1675, 1983.

ADAMS, D. S.; OLIVER, R. E.; AMEGHINO, E.; DEMARTINI, J. C.; VERWOERD, D. W.; HOUWERS, D .J.; WAGHELA, S.; GORHAM, J. R.; HYLLSETH, B.; DAWSON, M.; TRIGO, F. J.; MCGUIRE, T. C. Global survey of serological evidence of caprine arthritis-encephalitis virus infection. Veterinary Record, v. 115, n. 19, p. 493-495, 1984.

ADLER, H.; FRECH, B.; THONY, M.; PFISTER, H.; PETERHANS, E.; JUNGI, T. W. Inducible nitric oxide synthase in cattle. Differential cytokine regulation of nitric oxide synthase in bovine and murine macrophages. Journal of Immunology, v. 154, n. 9, p. 4710-4718, 1995.

AL-QUDAH, K.; AL-MAJALI, A. M.; ISMAIL, Z. B. Epidemiological studies on caprine arthritis-encephalitis virus infection in Jordan. Small Ruminant Research, v. 66, n. 1-3, p. 181-186, 2006.

ANDERSON, L. W.; KLEVJER-ANDERSON, P.; LIGGITIF, H. D. Susceptibility of blood-derived monocytes and macrophages to caprine arthritis-encephalitis virus. Infection and Immunity, v. 41, n. 2, p. 837-840, 1983.

ANUALPEC 2006: Anuário da pecuária brasileira. São Paulo: FNP Institute, 2006. 369 p.

BAIRD, G. J.; FONTAINE, M. C. Corynebacterium pseudotuberculosis and its role in ovine caseous lymphadenitis. Journal of Comparative Pathology, v. 137, n. 4, p. 179210, 2007.

BANNERMAN, D. D.; PAAPE, M. J.; LEE, J. W.; ZHAO, X.; HOPE, J. C.; RAINARD, P. Escherichia coli and Staphilococcus aureus Elicit differential Innate Immune Responses following Intramammary infection. Clinical and Diagnostic Laboratory Immunology. v. 11, n. 3, p. 463-472, 2004.

BANKS, K. L.; ADAMS, D. S.; MCGUIRE, T. C.; CARLSON, J. Experimental infection of sheep by caprine arthritis-encephalitis virus and goats by progressive pneumonia virus. American Journal of Veterinary Research, v. 44, n. 12, p. 23072311, 1983.

BÉLANGER, D.; LEBOEUF, A. CAE virus prevalence in a mixed goat herd. The Veterinary Records, v. 133, n. 13, p. 328, 1993.

BELLINGTON, S. J.; ESMAY, P. A.; SONGER, J. G.; JOST, B. H. Identification and role in virulence of putative iron acquisition genes from Corynebacterium pseudotuberculosis. FEMS Microbiology Letters, v. 208, n. 1, p. 41-45, 2002.

BIER, O. Microbiologia e Imunologia. Sao Paulo: Melhoramentos, 1984, 23 ed., p. 930-931.

BRINKHOF, J.; VAN MAANEN, C. Evaluation of five enzymed-linked immunosorbent assays and an agar gel immunodiffusion test for detection of antibodies to small rumminant lentiviruses. Clinical and Vaccine Immunology, v. 14, n. 9, p. 1210-1214, 2007.

BRODIE, S. J.; MARCOM, H. A.; PEARSON, L. D.; ANDERSON, B. C.; DE A CONCHA-BREMEJILLO, A.; ELLIS, J. A.; DEMARTINI, J. C. The effect of virus load in the pathogenesis of lentivirus-induced lymphoid interstitial pneumonia. Journal of Infectious Disease, v. 166, n. 3, p. 531-541, 1992.

CALLADO, A. K. C.; de CASTRO, R. S.; TEIXEIRA, M. F. S. Lentivirus of small ruminants (CAEV and Maedi-visna): review and perspectives. Pesquisa Veterinária Brasileira, v. 21, n. 3, p. 87-97, 2001.

CALLEGARI-JACQUES, S. M. Biostatistics: principles and applications. 1. ed. Porto Alegre: ARTMED, 2003. 256 p.

CARMINATI, R.; BAHIA, R.; COSTA, L. F. M.; PAULE, B. J. A.; VALE, V. L.; REGIS, L.; FREIRE, S. M.; NASCIMENTO, I.; SCHAER, R.; MEYER, R. Determination of the sensitivity and specificity of an indirect ELISA test for the diagnosis of caseous lymphadenitis in goats. Revista de Ciências Médicas e Biológicas, v. 2, n. 2, p. 88-93, 2003.

CETINKAYA, B.; KARAHAN, M.; ATIL,E.; KALIN, R.; De BAERE, T.; VANEECHOUTTE, M. Identification of Corynebacterium pseudotuberculosis isolates from sheep and goats by PCR. Veterinary Microbiology, v. 88, n. 1, p. 75-83, 2002.

CHAPLIN, P. J.; DE ROSE, R.; BOYLE, J. S.; McWALTERS, P.; KELLY, J.; TENNENT, J. M.; LEW, A. M.; SCHEERLINCK, J. P. Y. Targeting improves the efficacy of a DNA vaccine against Corynebacterium pseudotuberculosis in sheep. Infection and Immunity, v. 67, n. 12, p. 6434-6438, 1999.

CHIRINO-ZÁRRAGA, C.; SCARAMELLI, A.; REY-VALEIRON, C. Bacteriological characterisation of Corynebacterium pseudotuberculosis in Venezuela goat flocks. Small Ruminant Research, v. 65, n. 1-2, p.170-175, 2006.

COLOMBO, M. I.; BERON, W.; STAHL, P. D. Calmodulin regulates endosome fusion. Journal of Biological Chemistry, v. 272, n. 12, p. 7707-7712, 1997.

CORDEIRO, R. C. O Desenvolvimento econômico da caprinocultura leiteira. Revista do Conselho Federal de Medicina Veterinária, v. 4, p. 28-30, 1998.

CORTEZ-MOREIRA, M.; OELEMANN, M. R.; LILENBAUM, W. Comparison of serological methods for the diagnosis of caprine arthritis-encephalitis (CAE) in Rio de Janeiro, Brazil. Brazilian Journal of Microbiology, v. 36, n. 1, p. 48-50, 2005.

COSTA, L. F. M. Corynebacterium psudotuberculosis, the aetiological agent of caseous lymphadenitis in goats. Revista de Ciências Médicas e Biológicas, v. 1, n. 1, p.105-115, 2002.

CRAWFORD, T. B.; ADAMS, D. S. Caprine arthritisencephalitis: clinical features and presence of antibody in selected goat populations. Journal of the American Veterinary Medical Association, v. 178, n. 7, p. 713-719, 1981.

CUTLIP, R. C.; JACKSON, T. A.; LAIRD, G. A. Immunodiffusion test for ovine progressive pneumonia. American Journal of Veterinary Research, v. 38, n.7, p. 1081-1084, 1977.

CUTLIP, R. C.; LEHMKUHL, H. D.; SACKS, J. M.; WEAVER, A. L. Prevalence of antibody to caprine arthritis encephalitis virus in goats in the United States. Journal of American Veterinary Medical Association, v. 200, n. 6, p. 802-805, 1992.

DERCKSEN, D. P.; BRINKHOF, J. M. A.; DEKKER-NOOREN, T.; VAN MAANEN, K.; BODE, C. F.; BAIRD, G.; KAMP, E. M. A comparison of four serological tests for the diagnosis of caseous lymphadenitis in sheep and goats. Veterinary Microbiology, v. 75, n. 2, p. 167-175, 2000.

DESIDERIO, J. V.; TURILLO, L. A.; CAMPBELL, S. G. Serum proteins of normal goats and goats with caseous lymphadenitis. American Journal of Veterinary Research, v. 40, n. 3, p. 400-402, 1979.

DORELLA, F. A.; PACHECO, L. G. C.; OLIVEIRA, S. C.; MIYOSHI, A.; AZEVEDO, V. Corynebacterium pseudotuberculosis: microbiology, biochemical properties, pathogenesis and molecular studies of virulence. Veterinary Research, v. 37, n. 2, p. 201-218, 2006.

EAST, N. E.; ROWE, J. D.; MADEWELL, B. R.; FLOYD, K. Serological prevalence of caprine arthritis-encephalitis virus in California goat dairies. Journal of the American Veterinary Medical Associaton, v.190, n. 2, p.182-186, 1987.

EGGLETON, D. G.; MIDDLETON, H. D., DOIDGE, D. G.; MINTY, D. W. Immunisation against ovine caseous lymphadenitis: comparison with of Corynebacterium pseudotuberculosis vaccines with and without bacterial cells.
Australian Veterinary Journal, v. 68, n. 10, p. 317-319, 1991.

ELLIS, J. A. Immunophenotype of pulmonary cellular infiltrates in sheep with visceral caseous lymphadenitis. Veterinary Pathology, v. 25, n. 5, p. 362-368, 1988.

ELLIS, J. A.; HAWK, D. A.; HOLLER, L. D.; MILLS, K. W.; PRATT, D. L. Differential antibody responses to Corynebacterium pseudotuberculosis in sheep with naturally acquired caseous lymphadenitis. Journal of the American Veterinary Medical Association, v. 196, n. 10, p. 1609-1613, 1990.

ELLIS, J. A.; HAWK, D. A.; MILLS, K. W.; PRATT, D. L. Antigen specificity of antibody responses to Corynebacterium pseudotuberculosis in naturally infected sheep with caseous lymphadenitis. Veterinary Immunology and Immunopathology, v. 28, n. 3-4, p. 289-301, 1991.

ELLIS, J. A.; RUSSELL, H. I.; DU, C. W. Effect of selected cytokines on the replication of Corynebacterium pseudotuberculosis and ovine lentiviruses in the pulmonary macrophages. Veterinary Immunology and Immunopathology, v. 40, n. 1, p. 31-47, 1994.

ELNER, J. J. Tuberculosis in the time of AIDS: the facts and the message. Chest, v. 98, n. 5, p. 1051-1052, 1990.

FELDMAN, B. F.; ZINKL, J. G.; JAIN, N. C. Schalm's Veterinary Haematology. 5. ed. Philadelphia: Lippincott Williams and Wilkins, 2000. 1344 p.

FERNANDES, M. A. Caprine encephalitis arthritis: a contribution to the epidemiological study of dairy herds in the state of São Paulo. 1997. 70f. Dissertation (Master's Degree in Veterinary Clinic) - Faculty of Veterinary Medicine and Zootechny, University of São Paulo, São Paulo, 1997.

FLURI, A.; NENCI, C.; ZAHNO, M. L.; VOGT, H. R.; CHARAN, S.; BUSATO, A.; PANCINO, G.; PETERHANS, E.; OBEXER-RUFF, G.; BERTONI, G. The MHC- haplotype influences primary, but not memory, immune responses to an immunodominant peptide containing T- and B-cell epitopes of the caprine arthritis encephalitis virus Gag protein. Vaccine, v. 24, n. 5, p. 597-606, 2006.

FONTAINE, M. C.; BAIRD, G.; CONNOR, K. M.; RUDGE, K.; SALES, J.; DONACHIE, W. Vaccination confers protection of sheep against infection with a virulent United Kingdom strain of Corynebacterium pseudotuberculosis. Vaccine, v. 24, n. 33-34, p. 5986-5996, 2006.

GATES, N. L.; EVERSON, D. O.; HULET, C. V. Effects of thin ewe syndrome on reproductive efficiency. Journal of the American Veterinary Medical Association, v. 171, n. 12, p. 1266-1267, 1977.

GENDELMAN, H. E.; NARAYAN, O.; KENNEDY-STOSKOPF, S.; KENNEDY, P. G. E.; GHOTBI, Z.; CLEMENTS, J. E.; STANLEY, J.; PEZESHKPOUR, G. Tropism of sheep lentiviruses for monocytes: susceptibility to infection and virus gene

expression increase during maturation of monocyte to macrophages. Journal of Virology, v. 58, n. 1, p. 67-74, 1986.

GOLLNICK N. S.; MITCHELL R. M.; BAUMGART, M.; JANAGAMA, H. K.; SCREVATSAN, S.; SCHUKKEN, Y. H. Survival of Mycobacterium avium subsp. paratuberculosis in bovine monocyte-derived macrophages is not affected by host infection status but depends on the infecting bacterial genotype. Veterinary Immunology and Immunopathology, v. 120, n. 3, p. 93-105, 2007.

GORDON, S. The macrophage: past, present and the future. European Journal of Immunology, v. 37, p. S9-17, 2007.

GREWAL, A. S.; GREENWOOD, P. L.; BURTON, R. W.; SMITH, J. E.; BATTY, E. M.; NORTH, R. Caprine retrovirus infection in New South Wales: virus isolations, clinical and histopathological findings and prevalence of antibody. Australian Veterinary Journal, v. 63, n. 7, p. 245-248, 1986.

GUFLER, H.; GASTEINER, D.; LOMBARDO, D.; STIFTER, E.; KRASSNIG, R.; BAUMGARTNER. Serological study of small ruminant lentivirus in goats in Italy. Small Ruminant Research, v. 73, n. 1-3, p. 169-173, 2007.

JOHNSON, E. H.; VIDAL, C. E. S.; SANTA ROSA, J.; KASS, P. H. Observations on goats experimentally infected with Corynebacterium pseudotuberculosis. Small Ruminant Research, v.

12, n. 3, p. 357-369, 1993.

JORDAO, L.; BLECK, C. K. E.; MAYORGA, L.; GRIFFITHS, G.; ANES, E. On the Killing of mycobacteria by macrophages. Cellular Microbiology, v. 10, n. 2, p. 529548, 2008.

KAPETANOVIC, R.; NAHORI, M. A.; BALLOY, V.; FITTING, C.; PHILPOTT, D. J.; CAVAILLON, J. M.; CONQUY, M. A. Contribution of phagocytosis by Staphilococcus aureus activated macrophages. Infection and Immunity, v. 75, n. 2, p. 830-837, 2007.

KERR, M. G. Laboratory tests in veterinary medicine. 2. ed. São Paulo: Rocca, 2003. 436 p.

KLEVJER-ANDERSON, P.; ANDERSO, L. W. Caprine arthritis-encephalitis virus infection of caprine monocytes. Journal of General Virology, v. 58, p. 195-198, 1982.

KLEVJER-ANDERSON, P.; ANDERSO, L. W.; LIGGITT, H. D. Susceptibility of blood-derived monocytes and macrophages to caprine arthritis-encephalitis virus.
Infection and Immunity, v. 41, n. 2, p. 837-840, 1983.

KNOWLES JR, D. P. Laboratory diagnostic tests for retrovirus infections of small ruminants. The Veterinary Clinics of North America: Food Animal Practice, v. 13, n. 1, p. 1-11, 1997.

KNOWLES JR, D. P.; EVERMANN, J. F.; SHROPSHIRE, C.; VANDERSCHALIE, J.;. BRADWAY, D.; GEZON, H. M.; CHEEVERS, W. E. Evaluation of agar gel immunodifusion serology using caprine and ovine lentiviral antigens for detection of antibody to caprine arthritis-encephalitis virus. Journal of Clinical Microbiology, v. 32, n. 1, p. 243-245, 1994.

LAN, D. T. B.; TANIGUSHI, S.; MAKINO, S.; SHIRAHATA, T.; NAKANE, A. Role of endogenous tumour necrosis factor alpha and gamma interferon in resistance to Corynebacterium pseudotuberculosis infection in mice. Microbiology and Immunology, v. 42, n. 12, p. 863-870, 1998.

LARA, M. C. C. S. H.; BIRGEL JUNIOR, E. H.; FERNANDES, M. A.; BIRGEL, E. H. Experimental infection of goat arthritis-encephalitis virus in goats.
Archives of the Biological Institute, v. 70, n. 1, p. 51-54, 2003.

LARA, M. C. C. S. H.; BIRGEL JUNIOR, E. H.; GREGORY, L.; BIRGEL, E. H. Clinical aspects of goat arthritis-encephalitis. Arquivos Brasileiro de Medicina Veterinária e Zootecnia, v. 57, n. 6, p. 736-740, 2005.

LECHNER, F; VOGT, H. R.; SEOW, H. F.; BERTONI, G.; CHEEVERS, W. P.; VON BODUNGEN, U.; ZUBRIGGEN, A.; PETERHANS, E. Expression of Cytokine mRNA in Lentivirus-Induced Arthritis. American Journal of Veterinary Pathology, v. 151, n. 4, p. 1053-1065, 1997.

LEITE, B. L. S.; MODOLO, J. R.; PADOVANI, C. R.; STACHISSINI, A. V. M.; CASTRO, R. S.; SIMÕES, L. B. Evaluation of the occurrence rate of caprine virus arthritis encephalitis by the regional offices of the Agricultural Defence Office of the state of São Paulo, Brazil, and its mapping using a geographic information system.
Archives of the Biological Institute, v. 71, n. 1, p. 21-26, 2004.

LILENBAUM, W.; SOUZA, G. N.; RISTOW, P.; MOREIRA, M. C.; FRÁGUAS, S.; CARDOSO, V. S.; OELEMANN, W. M. R. A serological study on Brucella abortus, caprine arthritis-encephalitis virus and *Leptospira* in dairy goats in Rio de Janeiro, Brazil. The Veterinary Journal, v. 173, n. 2, p. 408-412, 2007.

MALIK, Z. A.; THOMPSON, C. R.; HASHIMI, S.; PORTER, B.; IYER, S. S.; KUSNER, D. J. Cutting edge: *Mycobacterium tuberculosis* blocks Ca^{2+} signalling and phagosome maturation in human macrophages via specific inhibition of sphingosine kinase. Journal of Immunology, v. 170, n. 6, p. 2811-2815, 2003.

McKEAN, S.; DAVIES, J.; MOORE, R. Identification of macrophage induced genes of *Corynebacterium pseudotuberculosis* by differential fluorescence induction. Microbes and Infection, v. 7, n. 13, p. 1352-1363, 2005.

McNAMARA, P. J.; BRADLEY, G. A.; SONGER, J. G. Targeted mutagenesis of the phospholipase D gene results in decreased virulence of *Corynebacterium pseudotuberculosis*. Molecular Microbiology, v. 12, n. 6, p. 921-930, 1994.

MENZIES, P. I.; HWANG, Y. T.; PRESCOTT, J. F. Comparison of an interferon-y to a phospholipase D enzyme-linked immunosorbent assay for diagnosis of Corynebacterium pseudotuberculosis infection in experimentally infected goats. Veterinary Microbiology, v. 100, n. 1-2, p. 129-137, 2004.

MEYER, R.; REGIS, L.; VALE, V.; PAULE, B.; CARMINATI, R.; BAHIA, R.; MOURA-COSTA, L.; SCHAER, R.; NASCIMENTO, I.; FREIRE, S. In vitro IFN- gamma production by goat blood cells after stimulation with somatic and secreted Corynebacterium pseudotuberculosis antigens. Veterinary Immunology and Immunopathology, v. 107, n. 3-4, p. 249-254, 2005.

MUELLER, P.; PIETERS, J. Modulation of macrophage antimicrobial mechanisms by pathogenic mycobacteria. Immunobiology, v. 211, n. 6-8, p. 549-556, 2006.

MYONES, B. L.; DALZELL, J. G.; HOGG, N.; ROSS, G. D. Neutrophil and monocyte cell surface p150.95 has iC3b-receptor (CR4) activity resembling CR3. The Journal of Clinical Investigation, v. 82, n. 2, p. 640-651, 1988.

NARAYAN, O.; CORK, L. C. Lentiviral diseases of sheep and goats: chronic pneumonia, leukoencephalomyelitis and arthritis. Review of Infectious Diseases, v. 7, n. 1, p. 89-98, 1985.

NOZAKI, C. N.; FARIA, M. A. R.; MACHADO, T. M. M. Surgical removal of caseous lymphadenitis abscesses in goats. Arquivos do Instituto Biológico, v. 67, n. 2, p. 187-189, 2000.

ovine caseous lymphadenitis. Journal of Comparative Pathology, v. 137, n. 4, p. 179210, 2007.

PANCHOLI, P.; MIRZA, A.; BHARDWAJ, N.; STEINMAN, R. M. Sequestration from immune $CD4^+$ T cells of mycobacteria growing in human macrophage. Science, v. 260, n. 5110, p. 984-986, 1993.

PATON, M. W.; MERCY, A. R.; WILKINSON, F. C.; GARDNER, J. J.; SUTHERLAND, S. S.; ELLIS, T. M. The effects of caseous lymphadenitis on wool production and bodyweight in young sheep. Australian Veterinary Journal, v. 65, n. 4, p.117-119, 1998.

PAULE, B. J. A.; AZEVEDO, V.; REGIS, L. F.; CARMINATI, R.; BAHIA, C. R.; VALE, V. L. C.; MOURA-COSTA, L. F.; FREIRE, S. M.; NASCIMENTO, I.; SCHAER, R.; GOES, A. M.; MEYER, R. Experimental Corynebacterium *pseudotuberculosis* primary infection in goats: kinetics of IgG and interferon -y production, IgG avidity and recognition by Western blotting. Veterinary Immunology and Immunopathology, v. 96, n. 3-4, p. 129-139, 2003.

PEPIN, M.; FONTAINE, J. J.; PARDON, P.; MARLY, J.; PARODI, A. L. Histopathology of the early phase during experimental *Corynebacterium*

Veterinary Microbiology, v. 29, n. 2, p. 123134, 1991.

PEPIN, M.; SEOW, H. F.; CORNER, L.; ROTHEL, J. S.; HODGSON, A. L. M.; WOOD, P. R. Cytokine gene expression in sheep following experimental infection with various strains of Corynebacterium pseudotuberculosis differing in virulence.
Veterinary Research, v. 28, n. 2, p.149-163, 1997.

PICK, E.; KEISARI, Y. A simple colorimetric method for the measurement of hydrogen peroxide produced by cells in culture. Journal of Immunological Methods, v. 38, n. 1-2, p. 161-70, 1980.

PICK, E.; MIZEL, D. Rapid microassays for measurement of superoxide and hydrogen peroxide production by macrophages in culture using an automatic enzyme immunoassay reader. Journal of Immunological Methods, v. 46, n. 2, p. 211-226, 1981.

PIETERS, J., Entry and survival of pathogenic mycobacteria in macrophages. Microbes and Infection, v. 3, n. 3, p. 249-255, 2001.

PINHEIRO, R. P.; GOUVEIA, A. M. G.; ALVES, F. S. F. Prevalence of caprine encephalitis virus infection in the state of Ceará, Brazil. Ciência Rural, v. 31, n. 3, p. 449-454, 2001.

PLÚDEMANN, A.; MUKHOPADHYAY, S.; GORDON, S. The interaction of macrophages receptors with bacterial ligands. Expert Reviews in Molecular Medicine. v. 8, n. 28, p. 1-25, 2006.

PRESCOTT, J. F.; MNZIES, P. I.; HWANG, Y-T. An interferon-gamma assay for diagnosis of Corynebacterium pseudotuberculosis infection in adult sheep from a research flock. Veterinary Microbiology, v. 88, n. 3, p. 287-297, 2002.

QUINN, P. J.; MARKEY, B. K.; CARTER, M. E.; DONNELLY, W. J.; LEONARD, F. C. Veterinary microbiology and infectious diseases. 1. ed. Porto Alegre: Artmed, 2005. p. 67-70.

RADOSTITIS, O. M.; BLOOD, D. C.; GAY, C. C. Veterinary medicine. A text of the diseases of the cattle, sheep, pigs, goats and horses. 8. ed. London: Baillère Tindall, 1994. p. 652-655.

RAJAVELU, P.; DAS, S. D. A correlation between phagocytosis and apoptosis in THP -1 cells infected with prevalent strains of Mycobacterium tuberculosis. Microbiology and Immunology, v. 51, n. 2, p. 201-210, 2007.

RIBEIRO, M. G.; DIAS JUNIOR, J. G.; PAES, A. C.; BARBOSA, P. G.; NARDI JUNIOR, G.; LISTONO, F. J. P. Fine needle aspiration puncture in the diagnosis of

Corynebacterium pseudotuberculosis in caprine caseous lymphadenitis. Archives of the Biological Institute, v. 68, n. 1, p. 23-28, 2001.

RIBEIRO, O. C.; SILVA, J. A. H.; OLIVEIRA, S. C.; MEYER, R.; FERNANDES, G. B. Preliminary data on a live vaccine against caseous lymphadenitis. Pesquisa Agropecuária Brasileira, v. 26, n. 4, p. 461-465, 1991.

RIBEIRO, O. C.; SILVA, J. A. H.; PEREIRA FILHO, M. Incidence of caseous lymphadenitis in semi-arid Bahia. Revista Brasileira de Medicina Veterinária, v. 10, n. 2, p. 23-24, 1988.

RIVAS, A. L.; TADEVOSYAN, R.; QUIMBY, F. W.; COKSAYGAN, T.; LEIN, D. H. Identification of subpopulations of bovine mammary-gland phagocytes and evaluation of sensitivity and specificity of morphologic and functional indicators of bovine mastitis. The Canadian Journal of Veterinary Research, v. 66, n. 3, p. 165-167, 2002.

ROSENFELD, G. Panchromic dye for haematology and clinical cytology. New combination of the May-Grunwald and Giemsa components in a single dye for rapid use. Memórias do Instituto Butantã, v. 20, p. 329-335, 1947.

RUSSELL, D. G. Mycobacterium tuberculosis: here today, and here tomorrow. Nature Review Molecular Cell Biology, v. 2, p. 569-577, 2001.

RUSSO, M.; TEIXEIRA, H. C.; MARCONDES, M. C.; BARBUTO, J. A. Superoxide-independent hydrogen peroxide release by activated macrophages. Brazilian Journal Medical Biological Research, v. 22, n. 10, p. 1271-1273, 1989.

SCHALM, O. W.; JAIN, N. C.; CARROLL, E. J. Veterinary haematology. 3. ed. Philadelphia: Lea & Febiger, 1986. 807 p.

SENTURK, S.; TEMIZEL, M. Clinical efficacy of rifamycin SV combined with oxytetracycline in the treatment of caseous lymphadenitis in sheep. Short Communications. The Veterinary Records, v. 159, n. 7, p. 216-217, 2006.

SILVA, E. R.; ARAÚJO, A. M.; ALVES, F. S. F.; PINHEIRO, R. R; SAUKA, T. N. Association between the California Mastitis Test and the Somatic Cell Count in the evaluation of caprine mammary gland health. Brazilian Journal of Veterinary Research Animal Science, v. 38, n. 1, p. 46-48, 2001.

SIMMONS, C. P.; DUNSTAN, S. J.; TACHEDJIAN, M.; KRYWULT, J.; HODGSON, A. L. M.; STRUGNELL, R. A. Vaccine potential of attenuated mutants of Corynebacterium pseudotuberculosis in sheep. Infection and Immunity, v. 66, n. 2, p. 474^79, 1998.

SMITH, M. C.; SHERMAN, D. M. (Ed.). Caprine arthritis encephalitis. Goat Medicine. Philadelphia: Lea & Febiger, 1994. p.73-79.

STABEL, J. R.; KEHRLI JR., M. E.; REINHARDT, T. A.; NONNECKE, B. J. Functional assessment of bovine monocytes isolated from peripheral blood. Veterinary Immunology and Immunopathology, v. 58, n. 2, p. 147-153, 1997.

TASHJIAN, J. J.; CAMPBELL, S. G. Interaction between caprine macrophages and Corynebacterium pseudotuberculosis: An electron microscopic study. American Journal of Veterinary Research, v. 44, n. 4, p. 690-693, 1983.

TESORO-CRUZ, E.; GONZÁLEZ, R. H.; SCHMID, R. K.; SETIÉN, A. A. Cross reactivity between caprine arthritis-encephalitis virus and type-1 human immunodeficiency virus. Archives of Medical Research, v. 34, n. 5, p. 362-366, 2003.

TING, L. M.; KIM, A. C.; CATTAMANCHI, A.; ERNST, J. D. Mycobacterium tuberculosis inhibits IFN-gamma transcriptional responses without inhibiting activation of STAT1. Journal of Immunology, v. 163, n. 7, p. 3898-3906, 1999.

TIZARD, I. R. Veterinary immunology: an introduction. 6. ed. São Paulo: Roca. 2002. 532 p.

TORRES-ACOSTA, J. F. J.; GUTIERREZ-RUIZ, E. J.; BUTLER, V.; SCHMIDT, A.; EVANS, J.; BABINGTON, K.; BEARMAN, K.; FORDHAM, T.; BROWNLIE, T.; SCROER, S.; CAMARA, E.; LIGHTSEY, J. Serological survey of caprine arthritis - encephalitis virus in 83 goat herds of Yucatan, Mexico. Small Ruminant Research, v. 49, n. 2, p. 207-211, 2003.

UNDERHILL, D. M.; OZINSKY, A. Phagocytosis of microbes: complexity in action. Annual Review of Immunology, v. 20, p. 825-852, 2002.

VAN HEYNINGEN, T. K., COLLINS, H. L., RUSSELL, D. G. IL-6 produced by macrophages infected with Mycobacterium species suppresses T cell responses. Journal of Immunology, v. 158, n. 1, p. 330-337, 1997.

VERGNE, I.; CHUA, J.; LEE, H. H.; LUCAS, M.; BELISLE, J.; DERETIC, V. Mechanism of phagolysosome biogenesis block by viable Mycobacterium tuberculosis. Proceedings of the National Academy of Sciences of the United States of America, v. 102, n. 11, p. 4033-4038, 2005.

VIANA, R. B. Influence of gestation, parturition and puerperium on the haemogram of goats ***(Capra hircus)*** of the Saanen breed, raised in the State of São Paulo. 2001. Dissertation (Master's Degree in Veterinary Medicine) - Faculty of Veterinary Medicine and Zootechny, University of São Paulo, São Paulo, 2001.

WALKER, J.; JACKSON, H. J.; EGGLETON, D. G.; MEEUSEN, E. N. T.; WILSON, M. J.; BRANDON, M. R. Identification of a novel antigen from Corynebacterium pseudotuberculosis that protects sheep against caseous lymphadenitis. Infection and Immunity, v. 62, n. 6, p. 2562-2567, 1994.

WALLIS, R.; ELLNER, J. Cytokines and tuberculosis. Journal of Leukocyte Biology, v. 55, n. 5, p. 676-681, 1994.

WEISS, D. J.; EVANSON, O. A.; DENG, M.; ABRAHAMSEN, M. S. Sequential patterns of gene expression by bovine monocyte derived macrophages associated with ingestion of mycobacterial organisms. Microbiology Pathology, v. 37, n. 4, p. 215-224, 2004.

WEISS, D. J.; SOUZA, C. D.; EVANSON, O. A.; SANDERS, M.; RUTHERFORD, M. Bovine monocyte TLR2 receptors differentially regulate the intracellular fate of Mycobacterium avium subsp. paratuberculosis and Mycobacterium avium subsp. avium. Journal of Leukocyte

Biology, v. 83, p. 48-55, 2008.

WERLING, D.; LANGHANS, W.; GEARY, N. Caprine arthritis-encephalitis virus infection changes caprine blood monocyte responsiveness to lypopolysaccharide stimulation in vitro. Veterinary Immunology and Immunopathology, v. 43, n. 4, p. 401-411, 1993.

WILKERSON, M. J.; DAVIS, W. C.; BASZLER, T. V.; CHEEVERS, W. P. Immunopathology of Chronic Lentivirus-Induced Arthritis. American Journal of Pathology, v. 146, n. 6, p. 1433-1443, 1995.

WILLIAMSON, L. H. Caseous lymphadenitis in small ruminants. Veterinary Clinics of North America: Food Animal Practice, v. 17, n. 2, p. 359-371, 2001.

WOO, S. R.; SOTOS, J.; HART, A. P.; BARLETTA, R. G.; CZEPRYNSKI, C. J. Bovine monocytes and macrophage cell line differ in their ability to phagocytose and support the intracellular survival of Mycobacterium avium subsp. paratuberculosis. Veterinary Immunology and Immunopathology, v. 110, n. 1-3, p. 109-120, 2006.

ZINK, M. C.; NARAYAN, O. Lentivirus-induced interferon inhibits maturation and proliferation of monocytes and restricts the replication of caprine arthritis-encephalitis virus. Journal of Virology, v. 63, n. 6, p. 2578-2584, 1989.

ZINK, M. C.; YAGER, J. A.; MYERS, J. D. Pathogenesis of caprine arthritis- encephalitis virus. Cellular localisation of viral transcripts in tissues of infected goats. American Journal of Pathology, v. 136, n. 4, p. 843-854, 1990.

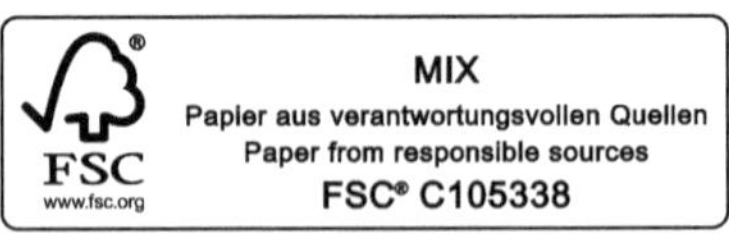

Printed by Books on Demand GmbH, Norderstedt / Germany